Registration Exam Questions III

Nadia Bukhari

BPharm, MRPharmS, FHEA, PG Cert Online Ed, PG Dip Pharm Prac, PG Dip Teaching Higher Ed

Clinical lecturer, Student Support Manager and Pre-registration Co-ordinator, UCL School of Pharmacy, London, UK

Naba Elsaid

MPharm, MPhil, PhD student

UCL School of Pharmacy, London, UK

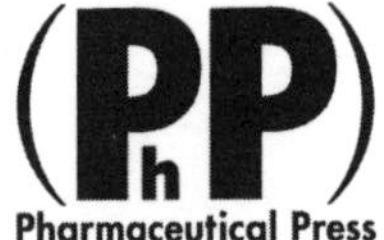
Pharmaceutical Press

Published by the Pharmaceutical Press

1 Lambeth High Street, London SE1 7JN, UK

Pharmaceutical Press is the publishing division of the Royal Pharmaceutical Society

First published 2014

Typeset by Laserwords Private Limited, Chennai, India
Printed in Great Britain by TJ International, Padstow, Cornwall

ISBN 978 0 85711 123 4

A catalogue record for this book is available from the British Library

Disclaimer

The views expressed in this book are solely those of the author and do not necessarily reflect the views or policies of the Royal Pharmaceutical Society. This book does *not* guarantee success in the registration exam but can be used as an aid for revision.

I would like to dedicate this book to my husband and my children – for all their love, support, encouragement and for their belief in me – Nadia Bukhari

I would like to dedicate this book to my guardian angel,
Zeeneh Elsaid – Naba Elsaid.

Contents

Preface

After the success of the first and second edition of *Registration Exam Questions*, a decision was made to write a third book with mostly clinical questions, testing the use and knowledge of the BNF and including a chapter on questions from the *BNF for Children*.

This book is a bank of just under 500 questions which are similar to the style of the registration examination. The questions are based on law and ethics, and clinical pharmacy and therapeutic aspects of the registration examination syllabus.

A new feature in this book is a chapter with 30 open book questions from the *BNF for Children*.

After completing four years of study and graduating with a Master of Pharmacy (MPharm) degree, graduates are required to undertake training as a preregistration pharmacist before they can sit the registration examination.

Preregistration training is the period of employment on which graduates must embark and effectively complete before they can register as a pharmacist in Great Britain. In most cases it is a one-year period following the pharmacy degree; for sandwich course students it is integrated within the undergraduate programme.

On successfully passing the registration examination, pharmacy graduates can register as a pharmacist in Great Britain.

The registration examination harmonises the testing of skills in practice during the preregistration year. It tests:

- knowledge
- the application of knowledge
- calculation
- time management
- managing stress
- comprehension
- recall
- interpretation
- evaluation.

There are two examination papers: an open book and a closed book paper. Questions are based on practice-based situations and are designed to test the thinking and knowledge that lie behind any action.

EXAMINATION FORMAT

The registration examination consists of two papers:

1 closed book (no reference material can be used): 90 questions in 90 minutes (1.5 hours)
2 open book (three specified reference sources permitted):
   - 80 questions in 150 minutes (2.5 hours)
   - 60 non-calculation-style (recommended time for these 1.5 hours)
   - 20 calculation-style (recommended time 1 hour).

The calculation-style questions are grouped together as a section of the paper.

The reference sources that the General Pharmaceutical Council permit for the registration examination are:

- *British National Formulary*
- *BNF for Children*
- *Medicines, Ethics and Practice 37*

The registration examination is crucial for pharmacy graduates wishing to register in Great Britain.

Preparation is the key. This book cannot guarantee that you pass the registration examination; however, it can help you to practise the clinical pharmacy and law and ethics questions, all very important aspects of the registration examination, and, as they say, 'practice makes perfect'.

Good luck with the examination.

Nadia Bukhari, Naba Elsaid
January 2014

Acknowledgements

The authors wish to acknowledge the support received from students and colleagues at the UCL School of Pharmacy, University of London. Nadia Bukhari would like to additionally thank Oksana Pyzik, from the UCL School of Pharmacy, for her contribution and help during the writing of this book.

We especially thank our parents and family for their continuous support and encouragement.

We would like to express thanks to our editors at the Pharmaceutical Press, who have been very supportive, and especially to Christina De Bono and Erasmis Kidd, for their guidance.

About the authors

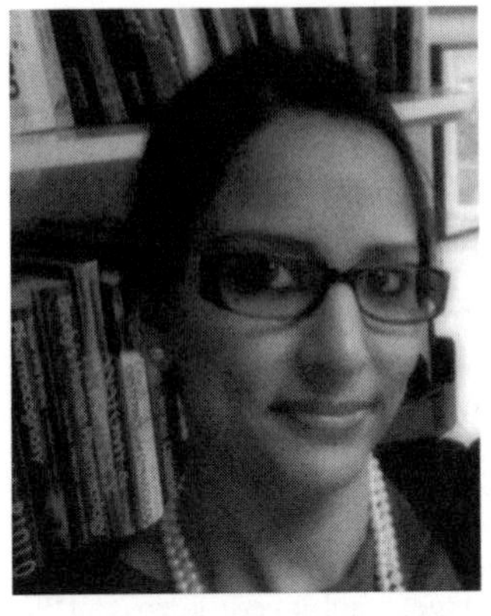

Nadia Bukhari graduated from the School of Pharmacy, University of London in 1999. After qualifying, she worked as a pharmacy manager at Westbury Chemist, Streatham, for a year, after which she moved on to work for Bart's and the London NHS Trust as a clinical pharmacist in surgery. It was at this time that Nadia developed an interest in teaching, as part of her role involved the responsibility of being a teacher practitioner for the School of Pharmacy, University of London. Two and a half years later, she commenced working for the School of Pharmacy, University of London, as the preregistration coordinator and the academic facilitator. This position involved teaching therapeutics to Master of Pharmacy students and assisting the director of undergraduate studies.

While teaching undergraduate students, Nadia completed her Post Graduate Diploma in Pharmacy Practice and her Post Graduate Diploma in Teaching in Higher Education. She then took on the role of the Master of Pharmacy Programme Manager, which involved the management of the undergraduate degree as well as being the preregistration coordinator for the university.

Since the merger with UCL, Nadia has now taken on the role of clinical lecturer, MPharm student support manager and preregistration coordinator for the university. She has a diploma in professional counselling and is a fellow of the Higher Education Academy. Nadia has recently taken on the responsibility of course coordinator for the final year of the MPharm.

Nadia will be leading the Professional Leadership module at UCL SoP, which involves designing, teaching and implementing the course to all four-year students studying the MPharm course. This module ties in well with Nadia's proposed PhD thesis which will be on 'Professional Leadership in Pharmacy Education'.

Nadia's interest in writing emerged in her first year of working in academia. Six years on, Nadia has authored four titles with the Pharmaceutical Press. In addition, she has taken on the role of sub-section editor for pharmacy and clinical pharmacology for the *British Medical Journal* for the onExamination publications. Nadia is also an MCQ question writer for the TP ONtrack, PJ Publications and Pharmaceutical Press.

Nadia has been chairing the Preregistration Conference and Study day at the Royal Pharmaceutical Society since 2012.

Nadia's 10 years of experience as a preregistration coordinator and clinical lecturer, coupled with the fact that she was a question writer for the registration exam for the RPSGB for four years, ignited her interest in private coaching for the examination. She has privately tutored many students, all of whom have given her positive feedback and have passed their exams at the first attempt after receiving coaching from her. For more information please visit her website: www.preregtuition.co.uk

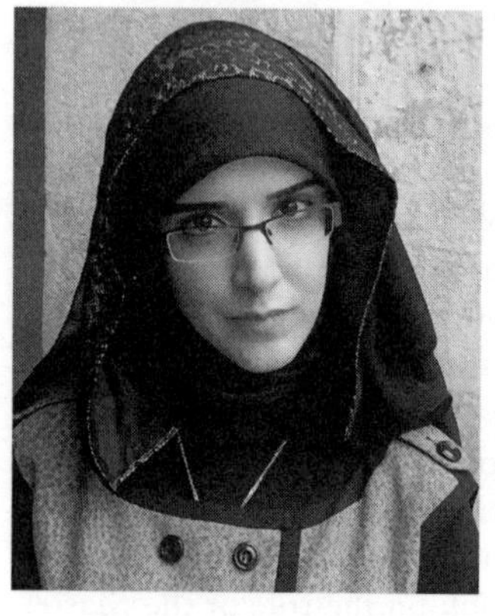

Naba Elsaid graduated from the School of Pharmacy and immediately took on a pharmacist manager role at one of Asda's busiest branches in 2009. She was awarded two prizes, for highest over-the-counter sales and maximum annual Medicines Use Review target, achieved across 199 branches in the UK. Naba worked for Excel Pre-reg, where she designed and helped to deliver a comprehensive programme for preregistration training pharmacists across the UK. The aim was to ensure that each student passed the exam with the knowledge, skills and confidence to excel in the field of pharmacy. Naba has delivered highly successful preregistration seminars at UCL School of Pharmacy and is publishing her second book in this series.

Naba is currently completing her PhD in Pharmaceutics at UCL School of Pharmacy and King's College Hospital in London. She has published articles and is currently a reviewer for *Investigative Ophthalmology & Visual Science* (*IOVS*).

Abbreviations

ACBS	Advisory Committee on Borderline Substances
ACE	angiotensin-converting enzyme
AV	arteriovenous
BMI	body mass index
BNF	*British National Formulary*
CD	controlled drug
CE	*conformité européenne*
CFC	chlorofluorocarbon
CHMP	Committee for Medicinal Products for Human Use
COX	cyclo-oxygenase
CPD	continuous professional development
CSM	Committee on Safety of Medicines
CYT	cytochrome
DNG	discount not given
DPF	*Dental Practitioners' Formulary*
EEA	European Economic Area
e/c	enteric-coated
eGFR	estimated glomerular filtration rate
GP	general practitioner
GP6D	glucose-6-phosphate dehydrogenase
GSL	general sales list
GTN	glyceryl trinitrate
HIV	human immunodeficiency virus
HRT	hormone replacement therapy
IBS	irritable bowel syndrome
IDA	industrial denatured alcohol
IM	intramuscular
IV	intravenous
IUD	intrauterine device
MAOI	monoamine oxidase inhibitor
MD	maximum single dose
MDD	maximum daily dose
MEP	*Medicines, Ethics and Practice Guide*
MHRA	Medicines and Healthcare products Regulatory Agency
MMR	measles, mumps and rubella

MR, m/r	modified release
MUPS	multiple-unit pellet system
MUR	Medicines Use Review
NHS	National Health Service
NSAIDs	non-steroidal anti-inflammatory drugs
OC	oral contraceptive
o.d.	omne die (every day)
o.m.	omni mane (every morning)
o.n.	omni nocte (every night)
OP	original pack
ORT	oral rehydration therapy
OTC	over-the-counter
P	pharmacy
PCT	primary care trust
PIL	patient information leaflet
PMR	patient medical record
POM	prescription-only medicine
POM-V	prescription-only medicine – veterinarian
POM-VPS	prescription-only medicine – veterinarian, pharmacist, suitably qualified person
PSA	prostate-specific antigen
PSNC	Pharmaceutical Services Negotiating Committee
q.d.s.	quarter die sumendum (to be taken four times daily)
RPSGB	Royal Pharmaceutical Society of Great Britain
SARSS	Suspected Adverse Reaction Surveillance Scheme
SLS	selected list scheme
SOP	standard operating procedure
SPC	Summary of Product Characteristics
SSRI	selective serotonin reuptake inhibitor
TCA	tricyclic antidepressant
TSDA	trade-specific denatured alcohol
UTI	urinary tract infection
WHO	World Health Organization

How to use this book

The book is divided into two main sections: open book and closed book.

Each section has four different styles of multiple choice questions, which are also used in the registration examination: simple completion, multiple completion, classification and statements.

SIMPLE COMPLETION QUESTIONS

Each of the questions or statements in this section is followed by five suggested answers. Select the best answer in each situation.

For example:
A patient on your ward has been admitted with a gastric ulcer, which is currently being treated. She has a history of arthritis and cardiac problems. Which of her drugs is most likely to have caused the gastric ulcer?

☐ A paracetamol
☐ B naproxen
☐ C furosemide
☐ D propranolol
☐ E codeine phosphate

MULTIPLE COMPLETION QUESTIONS

Each one of the questions or incomplete statements in this section is followed by three responses. For each question, one or more of the responses is/are correct. Decide which of the responses is/are correct, then choose:

A if 1, 2 and 3 are correct
B if 1 and 2 only are correct
C if 2 and 3 only are correct
D if 1 only is correct
E if 3 only is correct

For example:
A patient presents an FP10D to you.
Which of the below *cannot* be prescribed on this type of form?

1 ciprofloxacin
2 diclofenac
3 paracetamol

CLASSIFICATION

In this section, for each numbered question, select the one lettered option that most closely corresponds to the answer. Within each group of questions each lettered option may be used once, more than once or not at all.

For example:
Which of the following vitamins:

1 can cause ocular defects in deficiency states?
2 is necessary for the production of blood-clotting factors?
3 prevents scurvy?
4 can be used for the treatment of rickets?

☐ **A** vitamin A
☐ **B** vitamin C
☐ **C** vitamin D
☐ **D** vitamin E
☐ **E** vitamin K

STATEMENTS

The questions in this section consist of a statement in the top row followed by a second statement beneath.

You need to:

decide whether the *first* statement is true or false

decide whether the *second* statement is true or false

Then choose:

- A if both statements are true and the second statement is a correct explanation of the first statement
- B if both statements are true but the second statement is not a correct explanation of the first statement
- C if the first statement is true but the second statement is false
- D if the first statement is false but the second statement is true
- E if both statements are false

For example:

First statement

Microgynon is an example of a combined oral contraceptive pill.

Second statement

Combined pills contain oestrogen and testosterone.

The closed book questions should be attempted without using any reference sources, as you would for the examination.

The open book questions should be attempted with the GPhC's permitted reference sources for the registration examination, which are:

- *British National Formulary (BNF)*
- *BNF for Children*
- *Medicines Ethics and Practice 37*

Answers to the questions are at the end of the book. Brief explanations or a suitable reference for sourcing the answer are given, to aid understanding and to facilitate learning.

Important: This text refers to the edition of the BNF current when text was written. Please always consult the LATEST version for the most up-to-date information.

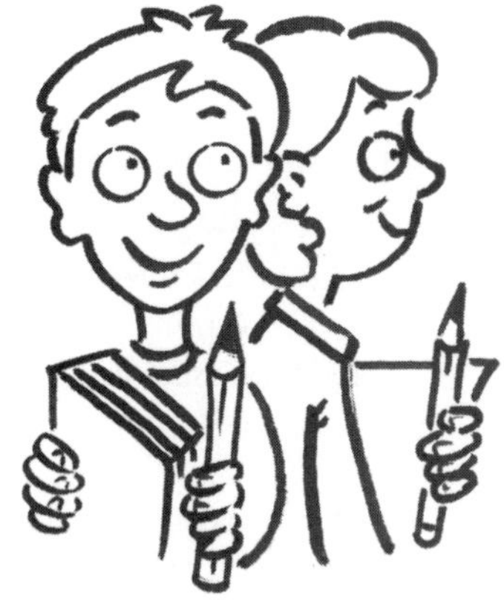

Open book questions

Nadia Bukhari and Naba Elsaid

SIMPLE COMPLETION QUESTIONS

Each of the questions or statements in this section is followed by five suggested answers. Select the best answer in each situation.

1 Mr K is a 59-year-old male who has recently been diagnosed with acute pyelonephritis. His GP decides to prescribe him a course of antibiotics. Which one of the following is suitable for treating Mr K's condition?

- ☐ A erythromycin
- ☐ B amoxicillin
- ☐ C doxycycline
- ☐ D gentamicin
- ☐ E ciprofloxacin

2 Liver toxicity can result from many drugs and is commonly associated with nausea, vomiting, abdominal pain, fatigue, dark urine and jaundice. Which one of the following drugs is not known to cause liver toxicity?

- ☐ A natalizumab
- ☐ B pioglitazone
- ☐ C methotrexate
- ☐ D calcium salts
- ☐ E tolcapone

3 Which of the following proprietary preparations is made by Organon?

☐ A *Tridestra*
☐ B *Norcuron*
☐ C *Caprin*
☐ D *Cystagon*
☐ E *Sofradex*

4 Miss J, a 27-year-old female, asks to speak to you regarding her hearing. She writes the following message and hands it over to you.
'My hearing has suddenly deteriorated but sometimes I hear "ringing sounds"?'
Which one of the following drugs is most likely to be attributed to this adverse effect?

☐ A metformin
☐ B cyclopenthiazide
☐ C azithromycin
☐ D cyanocobalamin
☐ E conestat alfa

5 You are giving a training session to preregistration pharmacists on antihypertensive drugs which affect the renin-angiotensin system. Which of the following drugs inhibits renin directly?

☐ A quinapril
☐ B lisinopril
☐ C telmisartan
☐ D aliskiren
☐ E valsartan

6 The use of all of the following should be avoided in patients with eGFR of less than 30 mL/minute/1.73 m^2, except which one?

☐ A eslicarbazepine acetate
☐ B moxonidine
☐ C anakinra
☐ D miglustat
☐ E pentoxifylline

7 Mr K is a 45-year-old male who has recently been diagnosed with tuberculosis. His GP decides to start Mrs K (Mr K's wife) on prophylactic therapy to prevent her from contracting her husband's infection. Given that Mrs K weighs 60 kg, which one of the following regimens is suitable for this indication?

- ☐ A ethambutol 900 mg daily for 2 months
- ☐ B pyrazinamide 1.5 g daily for 2 months
- ☐ C isoniazid 300 mg daily for 6 months
- ☐ D tetracycline 250 mg four times a day for 21 days
- ☐ E flucloxacillin 500 mg four times a day for 7 days

8 The local GP contacts you to ask for your advice. He says that one of his patients has recently developed colour blindness and asks you if this could be related to any of the drugs which she is taking? You check her patient medical record. Which one of the following drugs may be attributed to this adverse effect?

- ☐ A rifampicin
- ☐ B tranexamic acid
- ☐ C latanoprost
- ☐ D bendroflumethiazide
- ☐ E enalapril

9 Miss K comes into your pharmacy and asks to speak to you in private. She tells you that she has had 'bad breath' for a week now and that she has tried several remedies which have not helped. You search her medical record. Which one of the following drugs could be associated with Miss K's complaint?

- ☐ A *Microgynon 30*
- ☐ B salbutamol
- ☐ C disulfiram
- ☐ D mefenamic acid
- ☐ E glyceryl trinitrate

10 Which one of the following tablets is not scored?

- ☐ A *Cardicor*
- ☐ B *Mirapexin*
- ☐ C *Tenormin*
- ☐ D *Famvir*
- ☐ E *Hiprex*

11 Mr J is an 18-year-old diabetic patient on your ward. His glycosylated haemoglobin concentration is 8.0%. His consultant asks you how much this is in mmol/mol. Which of the following is the correct response?

☐ A 42 mmol/mol
☐ B 53 mmol/mol
☐ C 59 mmol/mol
☐ D 64 mmol/mol
☐ E 75 mmol/mol

12 Mr M, a consultant on your ward, notices that his patient with mixed colour irides has brown pigmentation and asks you if this could have been caused by any of their medications. Which one of the following could have caused this?

☐ A finasteride
☐ B flutamide
☐ C latanoprost
☐ D timolol
☐ E polyvinyl alcohol

13 Mrs F, is a 54-year-old female with hypertension. Her consultant wishes to give her an *Augmentin* injection and asks you how much sodium salt there is per 600 mg vial? Which of the following is the correct response?

☐ A 0.25 mmol
☐ B 0.5 mmol
☐ C 1 mmol
☐ D 1.35 mmol
☐ E 2.7 mmol

14 Which one of the following drugs is not known to cause gynaecomastia?

☐ A ethinylestradiol
☐ B estramustine
☐ C bumetanide
☐ D clonidine
☐ E bisoprolol

15 Which one of the following preparations contains 11.16 mmol of Na^+ per vial?

☐ A *Atriance* 50 mL vial
☐ B *Zovirax* 500 mg vial
☐ C *Tazocin* 4.5 g vial
☐ D *Kemicetine* 1 g vial
☐ E *Timentin* 3.2 g vial

16 Which of the following antibiotics is available in peach flavour?

☐ A *Augmentin* suspension S/F
☐ B *Noxafil* suspension
☐ C *Septrin* adult suspension
☐ D *Amoxil* paediatric suspension
☐ E *Rifadin* syrup

17 You are clearing out expired stock from the dispensary and find some loose black/grey capsules. Which of the following drugs are these likely to be?

☐ A *Neotigason*
☐ B *Galfer*
☐ C *Dalmane*
☐ D *Reyataz*
☐ E *Rocaltrol*

18 Which of the following is considered to pose a significant clinical interaction with candesartan?

☐ A aluminium hydroxide
☐ B alcohol
☐ C diazepam
☐ D ciclosporin
☐ E glyceryl trinitrate

19 Miss Z is a 26-year-old female. She has recently developed galactorrhoea. On questioning her, you find out that she has no children and no breast lumps, discharge or abnormalities. She has no changes to her medications. Which one of the following medications could have caused this?

☐ **A** omperazole
☐ **B** atorvastatin
☐ **C** captopril
☐ **D** cimetidine
☐ **E** mefenamic acid

20 Which one of the following is a modified preparation for theophylline?

☐ **A** *Natrilix* SR
☐ **B** *Nuelin* SA
☐ **C** *Flomaxtra* XL
☐ **D** *Betmiga*
☐ **E** *Emselex*

21 You receive a telephone call on Monday morning from one of your patients, Miss J, a 19-year-old diabetic female. She has obtained a new blood glucose meter '*Accutrend*' and asks you which strips are compatible for her device. Which one of the following will you recommend?

☐ **A** *Active* strips
☐ **B** *Aviva* strips
☐ **C** *Mobile* strips
☐ **D** *BM-Accutest* strips
☐ **E** *Breeze* 2 strips

22 All of the following preparations should be taken with or immediately after food, except which one?

☐ **A** posaconazole
☐ **B** ganciclovir
☐ **C** rufinamide
☐ **D** tenoxicam
☐ **E** pindolol

23 Which of the following preparations is not suitable for topical treatment of acne?

- ☐ A *Epiduo*
- ☐ B *Dalacin T*
- ☐ C *Zindaclin*
- ☐ D *Differin*
- ☐ E *Cutivate*

24 Miss N is a 4-month-old female who is due to receive her vaccinations. Which of the following vaccines is she scheduled to receive?

- ☐ A diphtheria (first dose)
- ☐ B measles, mumps and rubella vaccine, Live (MMR)
- ☐ C rotavirus vaccine (second dose)
- ☐ D human papillomavirus vaccine
- ☐ E tetanus (third dose)

25 Miss N is lactose and gluten intolerant. Which of the following liquids can she take?

- ☐ A *Fortisip* Yogurt Style
- ☐ B *Pro-Cal* Shot
- ☐ C *Fresubin* Energy Fibre
- ☐ D *Polycal*
- ☐ E *Fortimel* Regular

26 The administration of some drugs must never be stopped unless under the advice of the practitioner. This applies to all of the following drugs except for which one?

- ☐ A *Prestim*
- ☐ B *Keral*
- ☐ C *Aldomet*
- ☐ D *Tenoret*
- ☐ E *Visken*

27 Miss K is a 21-year-old female with severe acne. She presents with a small red bump around her nail that bleeds easily. Following examination her dermatologist states that it may be a periungual pyogenic granuloma. Which of the following preparations may be associated with this condition?

- ☐ A *Dermovate*
- ☐ B *Daktacort*
- ☐ C *Vectavir*
- ☐ D *Roaccutane*
- ☐ E *Nystaform*

28 Hypertrichosis is a local adverse effect of which one of the following *topical* preparations?

- ☐ A *Oruvail*
- ☐ B *Xepin*
- ☐ C *Daktarin*
- ☐ D *Gynest*
- ☐ E *Metosyn*

29 Which of the following consideration(s) is/are essential for the preparation of potassium chloride intravenous infusions?

- ☐ A avoid containers made from PVC
- ☐ B dilute in a large-volume infusion; mix thoroughly to avoid 'layering'
- ☐ C do not dilute
- ☐ D do not use non-rigid containers
- ☐ E prepared in pharmacy dispensary

30 Miss J is a 23-year-old female who reports to the A&E department with a cat bite on her right hand which she obtained two hours ago. Which of the following drugs may be given as a prophylactic measure to Miss J?

- ☐ A adrenaline
- ☐ B rifampicin
- ☐ C co-trimoxazole
- ☐ D trimethoprim
- ☐ E co-amoxiclav

31 Which of the following preparations can only be prescribed on an FP10D, GP14 or WP10D form if the prescriber has written 'ACBS' on the prescription?

- ☐ A loratadine syrup 5 mg/5 mL
- ☐ B cetirizine hydrochloride 10 mg tablets
- ☐ C *Duraphat* toothpaste 5000 ppm
- ☐ D *AS Saliva Orthana*
- ☐ E *Vectavir* cream 1%

32 Mr J comes into your pharmacy complaining of double vision. Which one of the following drugs could have caused this?

- ☐ A piroxicam
- ☐ B deflazacort
- ☐ C zolpidem
- ☐ D dicycloverine hydrochloride
- ☐ E dipyridamole

33 Mr T is a consultant on your ward. He asks for your advice on an antipsychotic which is equivalent in dose to fluphenazine decanoate 25 mg once every 2 weeks. What is your response?

- ☐ A haloperidol decanoate 25 mg every 2 weeks
- ☐ B haloperidol decanoate 50 mg every 4 weeks
- ☐ C flupentixol decanoate 40 mg every 4 weeks
- ☐ D pipotiazine palmitate 50 mg every 4 weeks
- ☐ E zuclopenthixol decanoate 20 mg every 2 weeks

34 Mrs K is a 43-year-old female who tells you that she felt 'faint' and fell after taking her medication. Which one of the following preparations is commonly associated with postural hypotension?

- ☐ A *Calcort* tablets
- ☐ B *NovoRapid* injection
- ☐ C *Rectogesic* rectal ointment
- ☐ D *Amikin* injection
- ☐ E *Mucodyne* oral liquid

35 In which one of the following circumstances is ciprofloxacin contraindicated?

- ☐ A myasthenia gravis
- ☐ B G6PD deficiency
- ☐ C epilepsy
- ☐ D quinolone hypersensitivity
- ☐ E a 9-year-old child

36 Which of the following preparations is only available for topical use?

- ☐ A ketoprofen
- ☐ B capsaicin
- ☐ C isotretinoin
- ☐ D griseofulvin
- ☐ E doxepin

37 You are a hospital pharmacist who is screening patient drug charts in the neurology department. Which of the following medications can be administered concurrently with paracetamol?

- ☐ A *Paramax*
- ☐ B *Tramacet*
- ☐ C *Midrid*
- ☐ D *Zamadol*
- ☐ E *Perfalgan*

38 Which of the following agents is not known to have a sedative effect?

- ☐ A promethazine
- ☐ B dexmedetomidine
- ☐ C midazolam
- ☐ D alcohol
- ☐ E azithromycin

39 Mrs K is a patient on your ward. She has a glomerular filtration rate of 49 mL/minute/1.73 m^2. Which of the following drugs should be avoided in this patient?

- ☐ A probenecid
- ☐ B metformin
- ☐ C acrivastine
- ☐ D balsalazide
- ☐ E prochlorperazine

40 Which one of the following preparations contains alcohol?

- ☐ A *Lamisil*
- ☐ B *Aldara*
- ☐ C *Canesten* HC
- ☐ D *Lucentis*
- ☐ E Simple Linctus, BP

41 Which one of the following drugs may colour bodily secretions red?

- ☐ A penicillin
- ☐ B metformin
- ☐ C danthron
- ☐ D triamterene
- ☐ E itraconazole

42 Which one of the following contains a potent topical corticosteroid?

- ☐ A *Fucidin H*
- ☐ B *Eumovate*
- ☐ C *Dermovate*
- ☐ D *Synalar N*
- ☐ E *Trimovate*

43 Which one of the following drugs can cause dry mouth?

- ☐ A digoxin tablets
- ☐ B ipratropium bromide inhaler
- ☐ C bumetanide tablets
- ☐ D aflibercept intravitreal injection
- ☐ E salmeterol inhaler

44 Mrs S is a 67-year-old female who has been admitted into the nephrology department with signs of acute renal impairment. Her medical records show the following drugs:

Paracetamol 500 mg capsules QDS PRN
Cordilox 120 mg f/c tablets BD
Persantin retard m/r capsules 200 mg BD
Naproxen 250 mg tablets BD
Benadryl Allergy Relief capsules 8 mg TDS

Which one of the above medications could have caused her kidney damage?

- ☐ A paracetamol
- ☐ B *Cordilox*
- ☐ C *Persantin*
- ☐ D naproxen
- ☐ E *Benadryl*

45 Which of the following side-effects is not likely to be attributed to allopurinol therapy?

- ☐ A rash
- ☐ B hepatitis
- ☐ C gynaecomastia
- ☐ D thrombocytopenia
- ☐ E hypotension

46 Which one of the following drugs has been associated with the development of Guillain-Barré syndrome?

- ☐ A cyclizine
- ☐ B allopurinol
- ☐ C streptokinase
- ☐ D olanzapine
- ☐ E metformin

47 Which one of the following drugs is not a calcium channel blocker?

- ☐ A felodipine
- ☐ B diltiazem
- ☐ C lercanidipine
- ☐ D isoniazid
- ☐ E lacidipine

48 Which of the following is an adverse effect of mannitol?

- ☐ A diarrhoea
- ☐ B incontinence
- ☐ C glaucoma
- ☐ D hypotension
- ☐ E hyperperspiration

49 Which of the following preparations contains 0.1% hydrocortisone?

- ☐ A *Canesten HC*
- ☐ B *Daktacort*
- ☐ C *Terra-Cortril*
- ☐ D *Calmurid HC*
- ☐ E *Dioderm*

50 When admitting patients with infectious diseases, doctors are required to notify the local authority for all of the following infections except for which one?

- ☐ A tuberculosis
- ☐ B diphtheria
- ☐ C leprosy
- ☐ D whooping cough
- ☐ E Lyme disease

51 Which of the following medical abbreviations is a form of cardiovascular disease?

- ☐ A CAM
- ☐ B CCU
- ☐ C NLM
- ☐ D CAD
- ☐ E SOB

52 To prevent relapse, undecenoate preparations should be continued for how many days after the lesions have healed?

- ☐ A 2
- ☐ B 3
- ☐ C 5
- ☐ D 7
- ☐ E 10

53 Which one of the following manufacturers produces *Convulex*?

- ☐ A Pfizer
- ☐ B Astra Zeneca
- ☐ C Pharmacia
- ☐ D Sanofi-Aventis
- ☐ E Roche

54 You are training counter staff on the different classes of laxatives and their products. Which of the following products is not a stimulant laxative?

- ☐ A *Dulcolax*
- ☐ B *Manevac*
- ☐ C glycerol
- ☐ D *Dioctyl*
- ☐ E *Fleet* Ready-to-use Enema

55 Which of the following drugs has an unlicensed indication in the treatment of neuropathic pain?

- ☐ A moclobemide
- ☐ B orlistat
- ☐ C amitriptyline
- ☐ D donepezil
- ☐ E clozapine

56 Mr J is planning to travel to the south-west regions of Kyrgystan for 7 days. His GP asks you to recommend antimalarial therapy. Given that there are no other contraindications. Which of the following therapies would you recommend?

- ☐ A chloroquine + proguanil hydrochloride
- ☐ B chloroquine
- ☐ C clindamycin
- ☐ D mefloquine
- ☐ E doxycycline

57 Which one of the following paracetamol preparations is not a black-listed item?

- ☐ A *Calpol* 6 Plus
- ☐ B *Panadol Capsules*
- ☐ C *Disprol* Soluble
- ☐ D *Medinol* Over 6
- ☐ E *Medinol* Paediatric sugar-free

58 The following gases can cause upper respiratory tract and conjunctival irritation, except for which one?

- ☐ A sulphur dioxide
- ☐ B chlorine
- ☐ C phosgene
- ☐ D nitrogen
- ☐ E ammonia

59 Which one of the following preparations does the following counselling extract belong to?
Drink within 2 hours of preparation. Avoid food, drink and other oral medications for 1 hour before and after dose administration

- ☐ A magnesium trisilicate
- ☐ B amoxicillin oral suspension
- ☐ C cholera vaccine
- ☐ D oral rehydration salts
- ☐ E *Zineryt* topical solution

MULTIPLE COMPLETION QUESTIONS

Each of the questions or incomplete statements in this section is followed by three responses.

For each question ONE or MORE of the responses is/are correct. Decide which of the responses is/are correct, then choose:

A if 1, 2 and 3 are correct
B if 1 and 2 only are correct
C if 2 and 3 only are correct
D if 1 only is correct
E if 3 only is correct

Summary				
A	B	C	D	E
1, 2, 3	1, 2 only	2, 3 only	1 only	3 only

1 Which of the following medicines are used in gastro-intestinal ulcer healing?

☐ 1 ranitidine
☐ 2 misoprostol
☐ 3 loperamide

2 Antacids may decrease the absorption in which of the following medicines when taken at the same time?

☐ 1 sucralfate
☐ 2 ranitidine
☐ 3 cimetidine

3 Aluminium hydroxide may cause:

☐ 1 constipation
☐ 2 alkalosis
☐ 3 diarrhoea

4 Which of the following medicines are contraindicated in pregnant women?

☐ 1 heparin
☐ 2 *Lipitor*
☐ 3 methotrexate

5 Which of the following drugs may be used in the management of chronic stable angina without left ventricular dysfunction?

☐ 1 verapamil
☐ 2 atenolol
☐ 3 glyceryl trinitrate

6 Identify the correct statement(s) regarding heparin.

☐ 1 Inhibition of aldosterone secretion by unfractionated or low molecular weight heparin can result in hyperkalaemia.
☐ 2 Unfractionated heparin has a long duration of action.
☐ 3 It is contraindicated in pregnancy.

7 Identify the correct statement(s) regarding fibrates.

☐ 1 Fibrates are first line therapy in patients who cannot tolerate a statin or who have a serum triglyceride concentration that is greater than 10 mmol/L.
☐ 2 Gemfibrozil and statins should not be used concomitantly.
☐ 3 Gemfibrozil is mostly used in men.

8 Side-effects including photosensitivity or phototoxic reactions may occur when taking which of the following drugs?

☐ 1 amiodarone
☐ 2 ofloxacin
☐ 3 leflunomide

9 What should be recommended for the treatment of severe acute asthma?

☐ 1 salbutamol
☐ 2 prednisolone
☐ 3 high flow oxygen

10 Sumatriptan should be used with caution when:

☐ 1 the patient is elderly
☐ 2 the patient has a history of angina
☐ 3 the patient has suffered from an MI previously.

11 Which anticonvulsive agent may cause Steven Johnson's syndrome?

☐ 1 topiramate
☐ 2 lamotrigine
☐ 3 valproic acid

12 Which of the following are examples of SNRIs?

☐ 1 venlafaxine
☐ 2 duloxetine
☐ 3 fluvoxamine

13 CNS stimulants are indicated for:

☐ 1 excessive sleepiness associated with narcolepsy
☐ 2 obesity
☐ 3 depression

14 Which of the following statements regarding Ménière's disease is/are true?

☐ 1 It is a vestibular disorder associated with nausea, vertigo, tinnitus and loss of hearing.
☐ 2 It may be treated with betahistine.
☐ 3 It may be treated with a diuretic alone or in combination with salt restriction and phenothiazines such as prochlorperazine.

15 A patient taking a TCA, an antihistamine and an antipsychotic may develop which of the following adverse effects?

☐ 1 dry mouth
☐ 2 CNS toxicity
☐ 3 tachycardia

16 An MAOI may be administered concomitantly with:

☐ 1 a benzodiazepine
☐ 2 a sympathomimetic
☐ 3 another MAOI

17 Which of the following antibiotics may cause severe haematological side-effects?

- □ 1 aminoglycosides
- □ 2 vancomycin
- □ 3 chloramphenicol

18 Side-effects associated with macrolide antibiotics include:

- □ 1 QT interval prolongation
- □ 2 reversible hearing loss with tinnitus
- □ 3 Stevens-Johnson syndrome

19 Identify the correct statements regarding ampicillin.

- □ 1 It is structurally related to amoxicillin
- □ 2 Less than half the dose is absorbed when given orally and absorption is further decreased by the presence of food in the gut.
- □ 3 It is well excreted in the bile and urine.

20 Which antibiotic(s) may be used to treat pseudomembranous colitis associated with C. *difficile* diarrhoea?

- □ 1 metronidazole
- □ 2 vancomycin
- □ 3 gentamicin

21 Rectal bleeding is a symptom of which of the following conditions?

- □ 1 irritable bowel syndrome
- □ 2 ulcerative colitis
- □ 3 haemorrhoids

22 Neuraminidase inhibitors like oseltamivir and zanamivir are indicated for:

- □ 1 prophylaxis of influenza A and B
- □ 2 post-exposure prophylaxis of influenza A only
- □ 3 post-exposure prophylaxis and treatment of influenza A and B.

23 A patient with a sulfa allergy may take which of the following medicines?

☐ 1 metoclopramide
☐ 2 gliclazide
☐ 3 sulfamethoxazole

24 Identify the correct treatment for chicken pox.

☐ 1 Neonates with chicken pox should be treated with a parenteral antiviral.
☐ 2 Children between 1 month and 12 years, who are otherwise healthy, do not require antiviral therapy.
☐ 3 Pregnant women do not require treatment.

25 Which of the following statements describe the mechanism of action of acarbose?

☐ 1 It inhibits alpha glycosidase intestinal enzymes.
☐ 2 It decreases absorption of starch and sucrose.
☐ 3 It delays the digestion of disaccharides and controls postprandial glucose level.

26 Which of the following may be used to treat vaginal and vulval candidiasis?

☐ 1 clotrimazole
☐ 2 ketoconazole
☐ 3 fluconazole

27 Concomitant use of gemeprost with mifepristone:

☐ 1 is contraindicated.
☐ 2 requires monitoring of blood pressure and pulse for 3 hours.
☐ 3 is used to induce abortion.

28 Atobisan:

☐ 1 is an oxytocin receptor agonist.
☐ 2 is licensed for the inhibition of uncomplicated premature labour between 24 and 33 weeks.
☐ 3 may be preferred to a beta 2 agonist because it has fewer side-effects.

29 Interferon beta:

- ☐ 1 is licensed for use in patients with relapsing, remitting multiple sclerosis.
- ☐ 2 is not recommended by NICE guidance.
- ☐ 3 may be administered orally or parenterally.

30 Medicines that may induce pancreatitis include:

- ☐ 1 sodium valproate
- ☐ 2 azathioprine
- ☐ 3 tetracycline

31 Neuropathic pain may be associated with:

- ☐ 1 chronic excessive alcohol intake
- ☐ 2 chemotherapy
- ☐ 3 HIV infection

32 Calcitriol:

- ☐ 1 patients should have their plasma calcium checked at intervals and whenever nausea and vomiting occur.
- ☐ 2 is a hydroxylated vitamin D derivative.
- ☐ 3 is licensed for the management of post menopausal osteoporosis.

33 Which of the following tests should patients prescribed methotrexate for rheumatoid arthritis undergo?

- ☐ 1 liver function test
- ☐ 2 chest x-ray
- ☐ 3 full blood count

34 *Lucentis*:

- ☐ 1 is administered by intravitreal injection.
- ☐ 2 is licensed for neovascular (wet) age related macular degeneration.
- ☐ 3 is recommended for the treatment of visual impairment due to diabetic macular oedema.

35 Acanthamoeba keratitis:

- ☐ 1 is an infection of the dermis leading to necrosis.
- ☐ 2 is a painful sight threatening condition.
- ☐ 3 can be caused by use of tap water to clean contact lenses.

36 Identify the correct advice regarding the use of eye drops/ointment.

- ☐ 1 Avoid use of preserved contact lenses.
- ☐ 2 Apply ointment at night.
- ☐ 3 Apply drops morning and midday.

37 Verteporfin:

- ☐ 1 contains the excipient butylated hydroxytoluene.
- ☐ 2 requires activation by local irradiation using non-thermal red light.
- ☐ 3 is administered by a specialist.

38 Treatment of nasal polyps includes:

- ☐ 1 short term use of corticosteroid.
- ☐ 2 a corticosteroid which may be given systemically, via nasal drops or nasal spray.
- ☐ 3 nasal drops which must be instilled standing upright.

39 Identify the correct statement(s) regarding sympathomimetic drugs.

- ☐ 1 They are included in nasal preparations and may damage the nasal cilia.
- ☐ 2 They are included in decongestant preparations.
- ☐ 3 They cause hypertrichosis.

40 Psoriasis may be triggered by which of the following drugs?

- ☐ 1 lithium
- ☐ 2 chloroquine
- ☐ 3 NSAIDs

41 Plaque psoriasis:

- ☐ 1 is characterised by epidermal thickening and silver scaling most commonly found on the extensor surfaces and scalp.
- ☐ 2 occurs after a streptococcal throat infection and is more common in children.
- ☐ 3 emollients should not be used as adjuncts to other treatments.

42 Acitretin:

- ☐ 1 is a vitamin A derivative.
- ☐ 2 is teratogenic for up to three years after use.
- ☐ 3 is the least toxic systemic treatment for psoriasis in women of childbearing age.

43 Pneumococcal vaccination is recommended for which of the following individuals at increased risk of pneumococcal infection?

- ☐ 1 welders
- ☐ 2 patients treated with systemic corticosteroids for over one month
- ☐ 3 patients with a cochlear implant

44 Live vaccines may be contraindicated in individuals who are:

- ☐ 1 pregnant
- ☐ 2 immunosuppressed
- ☐ 3 over the age of 65

45 Vaccines may be delivered by which of the following routes?

- ☐ 1 orally
- ☐ 2 intramuscularly
- ☐ 3 intravenously

46 The immunisation schedule of Human Papillomavirus Vaccine for girls aged 13–18 is as follows:

- ☐ 1 three doses; second dose 1 month, and third dose 12 months after first dose
- ☐ 2 single booster dose
- ☐ 3 three doses; second dose 1 month, and third dose 4–6 months after first dose

47 When using the volatile liquid anaesthetic halothane:

- ☐ 1 it can be administered to a child over 1 month.
- ☐ 2 avoid out of hospital dental procedures for patients under 18 years.
- ☐ 3 monitor for severe hepatotoxicity.

48 Which of the following drugs shows teratogenicity?

☐ 1 methotrexate
☐ 2 isotretinoin
☐ 3 phenytoin

49 Which of the following medicines results in an increased sedative effect when taken with alcohol?

☐ 1 metformin
☐ 2 diphenhydramine
☐ 3 hydromorphone

50 Which of the following drugs can be given for the management of anaphylaxis?

☐ 1 epinephrine
☐ 2 chlorphenamine
☐ 3 hydrocortisone

51 Medicinal products particularly associated with anaphylaxis include:

☐ 1 blood products
☐ 2 vaccines
☐ 3 aspirin

52 Which of the following statements are true regarding lithium toxicity?

☐ 1 Dehydration and diarrhoea may increase Li^+ serum concentration.
☐ 2 Early clinical features are non-specific but severe lithium toxicity symptoms include seizures, change in heart rate, fluid retention.
☐ 3 Lithium toxicity can occur if serum level over 1.5 mmol/L.

CLASSIFICATION QUESTIONS

In this section, for each numbered question, select the one lettered option that most closely corresponds to the answer. Within each group of questions each lettered option may be used once, more than once or not at all.

Questions 1–10 concern the following drugs:

- A febuxostat
- B penicillamine
- C potassium bicarbonate
- D sodium aurothiomalate
- E ciclosporin

Which one of the above drugs:

1 is contraindicated in hypochloraemia?
2 is contraindicated in exfoliative dermatitis?
3 can be given as an initial dose of 2.5 mg/kg daily in two divided doses?
4 is used in gout?
5 has nervousness as a side-effect?
6 has the Goodpasture's syndrome as a side-effect?
7 has a serious interaction when given with a NSAID?
8 should be used with caution in the elderly?
9 has an unlicensed use in severe acute ulcerative colitis?
10 can be used in Wilson's disease?

Questions 11–20 concern the following drugs:

- A pergolide
- B piracetam
- C citalopram
- D temocillin
- E raltegravir

Which one of the above drugs:

11 is indicated for HIV infection?
12 is indicated for septicaemia?
13 should be used with caution with major surgery?

14 should be followed with a glass of soft drink when taking the oral solution?
15 is contraindicated in patients with a history of fibrotic disorders?
16 has compulsive behaviour as a side-effect?
17 is indicated for panic disorder?
18 can the oral drops of the drug be mixed in apple juice before taking?
19 is manufactured as the brand name *Negaban*?
20 when 4 drops are given is equivalent therapeutically to 10 mg of its tablet?

Questions 21–31 concern the following antibiotics:

A amoxicillin
B benzylpenicillin
C ciprofloxacin
D cefotaxime
E metronidazole

Which one of the above drugs is used to treat the following conditions?

21 campylobacter enteritis
22 endocarditis caused by enterococci
23 *Haemophilus influenzae* epiglottitis
24 bacterial vaginosis
25 *Clostridium difficile* infection
26 otitis media
27 sinusitis
28 periodontitis
29 meningitis caused by pneumococci
30 pneumonia: low severity, community-acquired
31 chronic bronchitis: acute exacerbation

Questions 32–41 concern the following extra precautionary labels:

A **Warning: Do not stop taking this medicine unless your doctor tells you to stop (8)**
B **Protect your skin from sunlight – even on a bright but cloudy day. Do not use sunbeds (11)**
C **Warning: This medicine may make you sleepy. If this happens, do not drive or use tools or machines. Do not drink alcohol (2)**
D **Do not take milk, indigestion remedies, or medicines containing iron or zinc, 2 hours before or after you take this medicine (7)**
E **Take with or just after food, or a meal (21)**

Match the extra precautionary label with the drugs below:

32 timolol
33 *Ursofalk*
34 *Isotrex*
35 doxepin
36 oxytetracycline
37 *Neurontin*
38 *Remedeine*
39 sodium aurothiomalate
40 valganciclovir
41 *Tarivid*

Questions 42–51 concern the following side-effects:

- **A** myocardial infarction
- **B** blood disorders
- **C** hypersexuality
- **D** optic neuritis
- **E** antibody formation

Match the side effects caused by the drugs below:

42 carbimazole
43 etravirine
44 propylthiouracil
45 methotrexate
46 penicillamine
47 oxcarbazepine
48 bromocriptine
49 ethambutol
50 lamotrigine
51 somatropin

STATEMENT QUESTIONS

The questions in this section consist of a statement in the top row followed by a second statement beneath.

You need to:

decide whether the *first statement* is true or false

decide whether the *second statement* is true or false

Then choose:

- A if both statements are true and the second statement is *a correct explanation* of the first statement
- B if both statements are true but the second statement is *not a correct explanation* of the first statement
- C if the first statement is true but the second statement is false
- D if the first statement is false but the second statement is true
- E if both statements are false

1 **First statement**

Cefadroxil can be given in pregnancy

Second statement

Cefadroxil is not known to be harmful to the fetus

2 **First statement**

Mebendazole is usually given as a single dose, but a second dose can be given after two weeks

Second statement

Re-infection with threadworms is very common

3 **First statement**

Interferon Gamma-1b can be given to children for severe malignant osteopetrosis

Second statement

For children with a body surface area of 0.45 m^2 a dose of 50 mcg/m^2 three times a week would be appropriate

4 **First statement**

Lifestyle™ brown loaf can be prescribed on the NHS for children with coeliac disease

Second statement

The prescription must be endorsed with the letters ACBS

5 **First statement**

Microgynon 30 can be prescribed for a 13-year-old child

Second statement

The Fraser Guidelines should be adhered to when prescribing contraceptives for this age group

6 **First statement**

Intravenous insulin can be used for neonates in intensive care

Second statement

A dose of 0.02 units/kg/hour would be appropriate

7 **First statement**

Creatine kinase should be monitored with daptomycin therapy

Second statement

It should be used with caution in severe hepatic impairment

8 **First statement**

Zolmitriptan is contraindicated in breastfeeding

Second statement

It is present in breast milk in animal studies

9 **First statement**

In certain situations ACE inhibitors should be initiated under specialist supervision

Second statement

This is true of patients with hyponatraemia

10 **First statement**

Risperidone should be used with careful monitoring in pregnancy

Second statement

Extrapyramidal side-effects have been reported in neonates when taken in the second trimester of pregnancy

11 **First statement**

Roflumilast is indicated in step 3 of the BTS guidelines

Second statement

It should be used as an adjunct to corticosteroid therapy

12 **First statement**

Haemolytic anaemia is a rare adverse effect of mefenamic acid

Second statement

Coombs' test can be used to diagnose haemolytic anaemia

13 Mr K is a 79-year-old male who has recently been diagnosed with unresectable malignant pleural mesothelioma

First statement

Pemetrexed and cisplatin may be used to treat this condition

Second statement

Pemetrexed activates thymidylate transferase

14 **First statement**

Malathion is an insecticide which may be indicated for the treatment of *Sarcoptes scabiei*

Second statement

Application of acaricides after a hot bath improves treatment efficacy

15 **First statement**

Sedating antihistamines have significant antimuscarinic activity and adverse effects

Second statement

Cyclizine should be avoided in patients with severe liver disease as this increases the risk of coma

16 Dr G from the local GP practice contacts you regarding modified release preparation for indapamide 1.5 mg tablets. He asks you to suggest a preparation

First statement

Indapamide is a thiazide diuretic

Second statement

Tensaid XL is a suitable preparation

17 **First statement**

Selenium is a mineral

Second statement

Prolonged parenteral nutrition can cause selenium deficiency

18 **First statement**

Low molecular weight heparins are eliminated more quickly than heparin in pregnancy

Second statement

Low molecular weight heparins have a lower risk of osteoporosis development compared with heparin

19 **First statement**

Notifiable diseases are infectious diseases which pose a risk to the public and must be reported to the Proper Officer

Second statement

Whooping cough is an example of a notifiable disease

20 **First statement**

Dopamine hydrochloride intravenous infusion can be diluted to a maximum concentration of 3.2 mg/mL

Second statement

Dopamine hydrochloride infusions are incompatible with bicarbonate

21 Miss B is a 25-year-old female who has just been prescribed *MigraMax* oral powder.

First statement

MigraMax oral powder contains aspirin

Second statement

The dispensed label for this prearation should have 'Contains aspirin. Do not take anything else containing aspirin while taking this medicine' written on it

22 **First statement**

Macrodantin contains nitrofurantoin 50 mg formulated as macrocrystals

Second statement

Macrodantin may colour the urine yellow or brown

23 You wish to provide a customer with the contact information for *Ametop* gel

First statement

Ametop gel is made by Smith & Nephew Healthcare Ltd

Second statement

The company's email address is questions@smith-nephew.com

24 **First statement**

Hylo-Care eye drops are used to treat scleritis

Second statement

Hylo-Care contains sodium hyaluronate 0.1%, dexpanthenol 2%

25 **First statement**

Prontosan gel is available as a 30 mL tube

Second statement

Prontosan gel contains the surfactant sodium dodecyl sulphate

26 **First statement**

Morphine hydrochloride is contraindicated in phaeochromocytoma

Second statement

Chlorphenamine taken concomitantly with morphine hydrochloride increases the risk of sedation

27 Ms K is a 43-year-old female on your ward. She is currently taking mercaptopurine. Her consultant is considering initiating her on mesalazine

First statement

Mercaptopurine is an antimetabolite

Second statement

There is a possible increased risk of Ms K developing leucopenia if these two drugs are taken concomitantly

28 Mrs K has been diagnosed with advanced adrenocortical carcinoma. She is prescribed mitotane.

First statement

Hypogonadism is a very common adverse effect of mitotane therapy

Second statement

Mrs K has a 1 in 10 chance of developing hypogonadism with mitotane therapy

29 **First statement**

Sleep disturbance is common in depressed patients

Second statement

The use of hypnotic agents in the elderly increases the risk of injury as a result of falls

30 **First statement**

Nurse prescribers can only prescribe medicinal preparations, under the NHS, which are listed in the *Nurse Prescribers' Formulary*

Second statement

Doublebase emollient shower gel can be prescribed on an FP10P by a nurse prescriber

31 **First statement**

An emergency supply on the request of a doctor can be made by the pharmacist provided the prescriber provides a valid prescription within 24 hours

Second statement

Phenobarbital can be supplied as an emergency supply under the request of a doctor for the treatment of epilepsy

32 **First statement**

VSL 3 is a nutritional supplement

Second statement

VSL 3 can be prescribed on an FP10 for the maintenance of remission of ileoanal pouchitis induced by antibiotics in adults

33 **First statement**

Prograf intravenous infusion is administered over 12 hours

Second statement

Prograf intravenous infusion is incompatible with containers made from polyvinyl chloride

34 **First statement**

Fresubin Soya Fibre is a 'lactose-free' product

Second statement

'Lactose-free' is described by some manufacturers as a formula which contains less than 0.1 g lactose/100 mL

35 **First statement**

BiNovum is a combined oral contraceptive

Second statement

There are 14 tablets of norethisterone 500 micrograms available per cycle in *BiNovum*

36 **First statement**

The interaction between propanolol and adrenaline is considered a potentially serious interaction

Second statement

Propanolol taken with adrenaline increases the risk of developing severe hypertension and bradycardia

37 **First statement**

Tramadol can cause dry mouth

Second statement

Dry mouth can be relieved by sucking ice

38 **First statement**

Obstructive jaundice can cause pruritus

Second statement

Pruritus in palliative care patients requires treatment with topical corticosteroids

39 **First statement**

Multiple-application eye drops which are used in hospital wards should be discarded two weeks after opening

Second statement

Eye drops used before a surgical procedure should be discarded and not used again following the procedure

40 **First statement**

An optometrist independent prescriber can request an emergency supply for his/her patient

Second statement

The pharmacist making the supply must ensure that an entry is made in the prescriptions book to include the name and address of the prescriber

41 **First statement**

Minoxidil may cause hirsutism

Second statement

Co-cyprindiol can be used in the management of hirsutism

42 **First statement**

Carbamazepine tablets BP can be prescribed on an FP10D by a dentist

Second statement

Dental prescribers can only prescribe medicinal preparations, under the NHS, which are listed in the *Dental Prescribers' Formulary*

43 **First statement**

Patients taking tropicamide eye drops should be warned not to drive until their vision has returned to normal

Second statement

Tropicamide eye drops are used to dilate the pupils

44 **First statement**

Nasal polyps are malignant growths in the nasal lining

Second statement

Nasal polyps can be reduced in size with short-term use of corticosteroid nasal drops

45 **First statement**

An emergency supply can be made in response to a dental prescriber

Second statement

A valid prescription which is issued by a dental prescriber who is registered in Cyprus is legally recognised in the UK

46 **First statement**

Temazepam is a long acting anxiolytic agent

Second statement

Temazepam 20 mg tablets can be prescribed by dentists

47 The following statements concern the use of emollient bath and shower preparations.

First statement

Hydration can be improved by soaking in a bath containing emollient bath additives for 10–20 minutes

Second statement

Extra care should be taken when using aqueous cream in the bath as it makes surfaces slippery

48 **First statement**

Lucentis is administered as an intravenous injection

Second statement

A minor suspected adverse reaction to *Lucentis* should be reported to the Medicines and Healthcare products Regulatory Agency (MHRA) through the Yellow Card Scheme

49 **First statement**

The risk of developing peripheral neuropathy with isoniazid therapy may commonly occur in patients who are malnourished or have chronic renal failure

Second statement

Vitamin B_1 may be given to prevent the development of peripheral neuropathy associated with isoniazid therapy in patients who are at risk.

50 On a trip to the beach, one of your friends gets stung by a jellyfish.

First statement

Portuguese man-o'-war is a type of jellyfish

Second statement

Apply an alcoholic solution to disinfect the area

51 Mr X is taking morphine sulfate 84 mg daily.

First statement

This dose is equivalent to *Transtec* '35' patch

Second statement

Transtec patches should be replaced weekly

52 **First statement**

A teratogenic agent is one which causes embryonic malformations

Second statement

Heparin is teratogenic

53 **First statement**

Calcium Resonium may be indicated in cases of potassium depletion

Second statement

Effervescent potassium tablets BPC 1968 contain chloride ions

54 **First statement**

Acute porphyrias are hereditary disorders of haem biosynthesis

Second statement

Certain drugs such as rosuvastatin must be avoided in patients who suffer from acute porphyrias as they can trigger an acute attack

55 **First statement**

Co-cyprindiol is a combined hormone contraceptive

Second statement

Co-cyprindiol can be used in the treatment of hirsutism

56 Mr K is a 24-year-old male who has contracted acute pyelonephritis. He has epilepsy but no known drug allergies.

First statement

A two-week course of ciprofloxacin may be suitable for this patient

Second statement

Quinolone antibiotics may induce convulsions in patients with or without a history of convulsions

57 **First statement**

Indapamide is a loop diuretic

Second statement

Thiazide diuretics inhibit sodium reabsorption at the beginning of the distal convoluted tubule

58 **First statement**

Cidomycin is available as an injection for the treatment of septicaemia.

Second statement

Sanofi-Aventis is the manufacturer of this proprietary formulation

59 **First statement**

Amiodarone injection must be avoided in neonates unless no safer alternative is available

Second statement

Benzyl alcohol present in injections has been associated with fatal toxic syndrome in preterm neonates

BNF FOR CHILDREN (BNFC) QUESTIONS

For questions 1–15

Each one of the questions or incomplete statements in this section is followed by three responses. For each question, *one* or *more* of the responses is/are correct. Decide which of the responses is/are correct, and then choose:

A if 1, 2 and 3 are correct
B if 1 and 2 only are correct
C if 2 and 3 only are correct
D if 1 only is correct
E if 3 only is correct

1 Which of the following is *not* licensed for use in children?

☐ 1 oxycodone
☐ 2 indometacin
☐ 3 naloxone

2 Which of the following is *not* licensed for use in children under the age of 1 year?

☐ 1 flumazenil
☐ 2 dantrolene sodium
☐ 3 ciprofloxacin

3 The use of drugs in children, infants and neonates requires special care and doses should always be calculated with care because:

☐ 1 of differing target organ sensitivity.
☐ 2 the risk of toxicity is increased by a reduced rate of drug clearance.
☐ 3 they have different body weight as fat % from adults.

4 Difficulties in adherence to drug treatment occur regardless of age but for children which of the following may be relevant?

☐ 1 difficulty in taking the medicine (e.g. inability to swallow the medicine)
☐ 2 unattractive formulation (e.g. unpleasant taste)
☐ 3 carers' or child's perception of the risk and severity of side-effects may differ from that of the prescriber.

5 Poppy is a 4-year-old girl suffering from asthma. Her father is concerned and speaks to you about how she is waking in the night more than once a week. Poppy is currently using salbutamol by inhalation. You give advice based on the current asthma management guidelines. Identify the correct statements regarding chronic asthma management for children below:

- ☐ 1 Maximum dose of salbutamol for child under 5 years old is one puff daily.
- ☐ 2 Add inhaled corticosteroid OR leukotriene receptor antagonist if salbutamol is needed more than twice a week or if night time symptoms occur more than once a week.
- ☐ 3 If patient shows a poor response to salbutamol and inhaled corticosteroid or leukotriene receptor antagonist then refer to respiratory paediatrician.

6 Which of the following is/are contraindicated with daunorubicin therapy?

- ☐ 1 severe arrhythmia
- ☐ 2 hepatic impairment
- ☐ 3 pulmonary infection

7 Which of the following is/are side-effects of cyclophosphamide therapy?

- ☐ 1 vomiting
- ☐ 2 pigmentation of nails
- ☐ 3 anorexia

8 When prescribing isoniazid for children which of the following is/are true?

- ☐ 1 It is contraindicated in renal impairment.
- ☐ 2 Liver function should be monitored in children with pre-existing liver disease.
- ☐ 3 Dry mouth is a known side-effect.

9 When prescribing olanzapine for children:

- ☐ 1 It may cause hypothermia.
- ☐ 2 It is not licensed for use in children.
- ☐ 3 A dose of 15 mg daily can be prescribed in 15-year-olds for the treatment of mania.

10 Summer is a twelve and a half-year-old child who is initiated on a dose of 75 mg phenytoin twice daily for epilepsy. Which of the following doses is/are appropriate to prescribe as maintenance therapy?

☐ 1 75 mg bd
☐ 2 100 mg bd
☐ 3 150 mg bd

11 Which of the following would be appropriate to prescribe for a 10-month-old child suffering with acute pyelonephritis?

☐ 1 co-amoxiclav
☐ 2 nitrofurantoin
☐ 3 ciprofloxacin

12 Which of the following is not licensed for use in children?

☐ 1 clotrimazole
☐ 2 liothyronine
☐ 3 vasopressin

13 Which of the following statements is/are true?

☐ 1 Children with Segawa syndrome are sensitive to levodopa.
☐ 2 Most hypnotics may cause a hangover effect in children.
☐ 3 Adrenaline may cause dyspnoea as a side-effect.

14 With respect to the prescribing of mycophenolate mofetil in children:

☐ 1 It can be given by mouth in combination with a corticosteroid and ciclosporin.
☐ 2 The tablets are lavender in colour.
☐ 3 Children and their carers should be warned to report any signs of infection or bleeding immediately.

15 Prophylaxis of migraine in children should be considered if they:

☐ 1 suffer significant disability despite being treated for migraine attacks.
☐ 2 suffer six attacks a month.
☐ 3 cannot take treatment for migraine attacks.

For questions 16–25

Each of the questions or incomplete statements in this section is followed by five suggested answers. Select the best answer from A–E in each case.

16 If abnormal losses of electrolytes are suspected, then faeces, vomit, or aspiration should be saved and analysed where possible. Where this is impracticable the approximations may be helpful in planning electrolyte replacement therapy. In children the approximate electrolyte content in gastro-intestinal secretions, in millimoles per litre, are:

☐ A

	H^+	K^+	HCO_3^-	Cl^-
Gastric	40–60	20–80	–	–

☐ B

	H^+	K^+	HCO_3^-	Cl^-
Gastric	40–60	5–20	–	100–150

☐ C

	H^+	K^+	HCO_3^-	Cl^-
Gastric	20–60	40–80	100–150	100–150

☐ D

	H^+	K^+	HCO_3^-	Cl^-
Gastric	–	40–80	–	100–150

☐ E

	H^+	K^+	HCO_3^-	Cl^-
Gastric	20–60	40–80	30–150	80–120

17 Which one of the following drugs is not licensed for use in children under the age of 12?

- ☐ A Bendroflumethiazide
- ☐ B Digoxin
- ☐ C Bumetanide
- ☐ D Iodine
- ☐ E Furosemide

18 Anagrelide is initiated under specialist supervision. Although it is not licensed for use in children, it is indicated for use in:

- ☐ A oedema in heart failure, renal disease and hepatic disease; pulmonary oedema
- ☐ B cytotoxic-induced neutropenia
- ☐ C following peripheral stem cell or bone-marrow transplantation
- ☐ D hyperphosphataemia in patients on haemodialysis or peritoneal dialysis
- ☐ E essential thrombocythaemia in at-risk children who have not responded adequately to other therapy or who are intolerant of it

19 A neonate less than 29 weeks postmenstrual age with a weight of 2 kg has been prescribed gentamicin (as a multiple dose regime by slow intravenous injection) to treat neonatal sepsis. What is the total daily dose?

- ☐ A 2.5 mg
- ☐ B 3.5 mg
- ☐ C 4.5 mg
- ☐ D 4 mg
- ☐ E 5 mg

20 A healthy one-year-old boy with a body weight of 9 kg has the following surface area (m^2).

- ☐ A 0.80
- ☐ B 0.18
- ☐ C 0.48
- ☐ D 0.46
- ☐ E 0.20

21 Identify the side-effects associated with the use of alprostadil, particularly in neonates under 2 kg.

- ☐ A apnoea
- ☐ B rash
- ☐ C interstitial nephritis
- ☐ D pancytopenia
- ☐ E hyponatraemia

22 All of the following statements regarding croup are true except?

- ☐ A Mild croup is largely self limiting.
- ☐ B Severe croup calls for hospital admission – a single dose of either dexamethasone 150 micrograms/kg or prednisolone 1–2 mg/kg, can be administered by mouth before transfer to hospital.
- ☐ C For severe croup not effectively controlled with corticosteroid treatment, nebulised adrenaline solution 1 in 1000 (1 mg/mL) can be given with close clinical monitoring in a dose of 400 micrograms/kg (max. 5 mg) repeated after 30 minutes if necessary.
- ☐ D The effects of nebulised adrenaline last 6–12 hours; the child needs to be carefully monitored for recurrence of the obstruction.
- ☐ E In hospital, dexamethasone 150 micrograms/kg (by mouth or by injection) or budesonide 2 mg by nebulisation will often reduce symptoms; the dose may be repeated after 12 hours if necessary.

23 Which of the following is the correct dose for proguanil used for the prophylaxis of malaria in a 6-year-old girl weighing 21 kg?

- ☐ A 25 mg daily
- ☐ B 50 mg daily
- ☐ C 100 mg daily
- ☐ D 150 mg daily
- ☐ E 200 mg daily

24 Which of the following is *not* a suitable *H. pylori* regime in children aged 4 years?

- ☐ A 250 mg twice daily amoxicillin + clarithromycin + omeprazole
- ☐ B 500 mg three times daily amoxicillin + metronidazole + omeprazole
- ☐ C 250 mg clarithromycin + amoxicillin + omeprazole
- ☐ D 100 mg twice daily metronidazole + clarithromycin + omeprazole
- ☐ E 100 mg three times daily metronidazole + amoxicillin + omeprazole

25 Which of the following is *not* an acceptable class of medicine that can be prescribed in children?

- ☐ A ACE inhibitors
- ☐ B thiazide diuretics
- ☐ C beta-blocker
- ☐ D loop diuretics
- ☐ E alpha blockers

For questions 26–30

For each numbered question, select the one lettered option that most closely corresponds to the answer. Within each group of questions each lettered option may be used once, more than once, or not at all.

Choose from the following options:

- A penicillin G
- B aciclovir
- C trimethoprim
- D baclofen
- E atenolol

Which one of the above drugs:

26 can be applied five times daily as the cream?
27 may cause interstitial nephritis as a side-effect?
28 may cause convulsions in high doses in the presence of renal impairment?
29 may be used in the treatment of pneumocystis pneumonia?
30 is contraindicated in blood dyscrasias?

Closed book questions

Nadia Bukhari and Naba Elsaid

SIMPLE COMPLETION QUESTIONS

Each of the questions or statements in this section is followed by five suggested answers. Select the best answer in each situation.

1 Which of the following drug combinations is known to introduce a risk of rhabdomyolysis?

- ☐ A ibuprofen with paracetamol
- ☐ B digoxin with amiodarone
- ☐ C beclometasone with theophylline
- ☐ D fluvastatin with bezafibrate
- ☐ E phenytoin with atenolol

2 Miss UY asks your advice on taking her combined oral contraceptive as she is 19 hours late in taking her next tablet. She is at the middle of her cycle. Which of the following would be the correct advice?

- ☐ A Take two tablets now and no further action is required.
- ☐ B Take the tablet straight away and no further action is required.
- ☐ C Take the tablet straight away and use other contraception for 7 days.
- ☐ D Take the tablet straight away and use other contraception for 14 days.
- ☐ E Stop the present cycle of the pill and start a new cycle in 7 days' time.

3 For which one of the following patients could you recommend sodium citrate sachets for the symptomatic relief of cystitis? (Assume that these patients are taking no medication other than that mentioned.)

- ☐ A a 45-year-old woman who is taking bendroflumethiazide
- ☐ B a 45-year-old man who is taking paracetamol
- ☐ C a 45-year-old woman who is taking levodopa
- ☐ D a 45-year-old woman who is taking lithium carbonate
- ☐ E a 25-year-old pregnant woman who is taking no medication

4 Which one of the following statements about supply of over-the-counter medicines is correct?

- ☐ A Hydrocortisone 1% cream is licensed for use in children of 8 years and over.
- ☐ B Naproxen 250 mg tablets are licensed for the treatment of dysmenorrhoea only.
- ☐ C Chloramphenicol 1% eye ointment is licensed for the treatment of conjunctivitis and styes.
- ☐ D Diclofenac 12.5 mg tablets are licensed for the treatment of muscular pain only.
- ☐ E Amoxicillin capsules are licensed for the treatment of tonsillitis.

5 Which one of the following herbal products should *not* be taken together with *Imigran Recovery* (sumatriptan) tablets?

- ☐ A agnus castus tablets
- ☐ B evening primrose oil capsules
- ☐ C ginseng tablets
- ☐ D passiflora capsules
- ☐ E St John's wort tablets

6 Which of the following should be given after food?

- ☐ A amoxicillin
- ☐ B naproxen
- ☐ C digoxin
- ☐ D lisinopril
- ☐ E temazepam

7 Mrs TG is suffering with motion sickness and comes to the pharmacy for some tablets. Which one of the following drugs is *not* licensed for OTC sale for the prevention of motion sickness?

- ☐ A cinnarizine
- ☐ B meclozine
- ☐ C prochlorperazine
- ☐ D promethazine hydrochloride
- ☐ E promethazine teoclate

8 Which one of the following is *not* a symptom of hypoglycaemia?

- ☐ A excessive sweating
- ☐ B feeling hot
- ☐ C pallor
- ☐ D palpitations
- ☐ E trembling

9 Which one of the childhood infectious diseases listed below is most closely characterised by the following symptoms?
Prodromal illness with fever, cold-like symptoms, conjunctivitis, cough, irritability, and small, greyish, irregular lesions surrounded by an erythematous base, occurring on the inside of the cheeks. These symptoms followed after 3 to 5 days by a maculopapular rash appearing first behind the ears, then spreading down the body, becoming confluent and fading by the third day.

- ☐ A chickenpox
- ☐ B impetigo
- ☐ C measles
- ☐ D meningitis
- ☐ E pneumonia

10 Mr CV has come to the pharmacy complaining of a tingling sensation above his lip. He suffers with cold sores frequently and would like something for it. You recommend penciclovir cream. How frequently should penciclovir 1% cream be applied for the treatment of cold sores?

- ☐ A twice a day
- ☐ B four times a day
- ☐ C five times a day
- ☐ D six times a day
- ☐ E eight times a day

11 Mr TH is taking GTN tablets for angina. Which of the following counselling points is false with regard to GTN tablets?

- ☐ A If the patient experiences chest pain, they should take a tablet immediately by putting it under the tongue.
- ☐ B GTN tablets should be discarded 8 weeks after opening them.
- ☐ C The tablets should preferably be taken standing up.
- ☐ D The tablets should not be transferred to another container.
- ☐ E Facial flushing may occur after taking the tablets.

12 Ms QW is taking regular dexamethasone. Which of the following is not a recognised side-effect of corticosteroid therapy?

- ☐ A weight gain
- ☐ B hypertension
- ☐ C osteoporosis
- ☐ D Addison's disease
- ☐ E diabetes

13 Steroid creams are routinely sold over the counter. In which of the following situations can hydrocortisone 1% cream be recommended over the counter?

- ☐ A in a 9-year-old child with an insect bite on the arm
- ☐ B for contact dermatitis on the neck line of a post-menopausal female
- ☐ C for acne on the back of a 14-year-old male
- ☐ D for the external treatment of chicken pox in an adult
- ☐ E for a patient who has tried it for 7 days and would like to continue for a further 7 days

14 Which of the following is a toxic effect of theophylline?

- ☐ A convulsions
- ☐ B watering eyes
- ☐ C drowsiness
- ☐ D bruising
- ☐ E goitre

15 Ms OP is a frequent migraine sufferer. Which of the following drugs on her PMR is known to commonly precipitate migraine?

- ☐ A metoclopramide
- ☐ B *Dianette*
- ☐ C diazepam
- ☐ D atenolol
- ☐ E ibuprofen

16 From the following scenarios, which one of the following patients would have to pay the NHS prescriptions charge?

- ☐ A a woman who has had a still birth within the last year
- ☐ B a 63-year-old woman on hormone replacement therapy
- ☐ C a patient with type II diabetes mellitus controlled by diet
- ☐ D a patient with epilepsy requiring continuous anticonvulsant therapy
- ☐ E a patient who currently receives income support

17 The recommended temperature range for a refrigerator is:

- ☐ A 0°C–4°C
- ☐ B 0°C–8°C
- ☐ C 2°C–6°C
- ☐ D 2°C–8°C
- ☐ E 4°C–10°C

18 Which of the following drug–side-effect combinations is correct?

- ☐ A amiodarone: slate grey skin
- ☐ B naproxen: gout
- ☐ C warfarin: vitamin D deficiency
- ☐ D diazepam: tendon damage
- ☐ E ciprofloxacin: black stools

19 Mrs TK has been started on furosemide. She is concerned as she has read on the internet that there are lots of side-effects associated with this medicine. Which of the following is not a property of loop diuretics?

- ☐ A may precipitate diabetes mellitus
- ☐ B may precipitate gout
- ☐ C may cause hypokalaemia
- ☐ D may cause hypermagnesaemia
- ☐ E may precipitate hyponatraemia

20 Mr UY is a regular alcohol drinker. He has recently been told by his GP to reduce his alcohol consumption as it is affecting his health. How many units of alcohol are recommended as a safe weekly limit for men and women to drink?

- ☐ A men 14 and women 14
- ☐ B men 21 and women 14
- ☐ C men 21 and women 21
- ☐ D men 28 and women 14
- ☐ E men 28 and women 28

21 Miss MB is taking aluminium hydroxide as she is suffering from indigestion. Intestinal absorption of which of the following drugs may be impaired when taken with aluminium hydroxide?

- ☐ A flucloxacillin
- ☐ B cefalexin
- ☐ C co-amoxiclav
- ☐ D tetracycline
- ☐ E vancomycin

22 Dr NV wishes to prescribe a beta-blocker for hypertension, for one of his patients, who suffers from various other medical conditions. The GP asks for your advice as she is unsure whether a beta-blocker would be contraindicated in this patient.
For which ONE of the following conditions are beta-blockers contraindicated?

- ☐ A diabetes
- ☐ B obesity
- ☐ C renal impairment
- ☐ D portal hypertension
- ☐ E asthma

23 Mr YF suffers with Parkinson's disease. He is prescribed procyclidine as he has been recently experiencing extrapyramidal side-effects associated with L-dopa therapy. Which of the following is *not* a side-effect of procyclidine?

- ☐ A urinary retention
- ☐ B constipation
- ☐ C drowsiness
- ☐ D blurred vision
- ☐ E bradycardia

24 Miss RF is prescribed warfarin tablets on admission to hospital. Which of the following is the correct indication for this drug?

- ☐ A gout
- ☐ B left ventricular failure
- ☐ C hypertension
- ☐ D atrial fibrillation
- ☐ E depression

25 Which of the following antibiotics, if taken orally, should be taken an hour before food or two hours after food?

- ☐ A flucloxacillin
- ☐ B amoxicillin
- ☐ C co-amoxiclav
- ☐ D metronidazole
- ☐ E clindamycin

26 Miss OU comes to your pharmacy as she is going to Malta and wants to buy a tanning lotion. You check her PMR and notice that one of her drugs causes phototoxicity.
Which of the following drugs may cause this effect?

- ☐ A propranolol
- ☐ B doxycycline
- ☐ C lisinopril
- ☐ D simvastatin
- ☐ E lactulose

<table>
<tr><td>Pharmacy stamp</td><td>Age

65</td><td rowspan="2">Name (including forename) and address

M Turmeric

56 Chillie Street</td></tr>
<tr><td>Number of days' treatment

N.B. Ensure dose is stated</td><td></td></tr>
<tr><td>Endorsements</td><td>Warfarin 3mg
MDU (28)</td><td rowspan="3">Office use</td></tr>
<tr><td>Signature of doctor

Nadia Bukhari</td><td>27 April 2012

Balmoral Surgery

Balmoral Road

Surbiton KT5</td></tr>
<tr><td>NHS</td><td>PATIENTS – please read the notes overleaf</td></tr>
</table>

27 Assuming today's date is 4 June 2013, the above prescription is not valid because:

- ☐ A the patient's date of birth is missing
- ☐ B the patient's postcode is missing
- ☐ C the number of days' treatment is missing
- ☐ D the prescription has expired
- ☐ E the direction for taking the medication is missing

Pharmacy stamp	Age 35	Name (including forename) and address D Berry 98 Capital Road London W1
Number of days' treatment N.B. Ensure dose is stated		
Endorsements	MST 20mg Take one as directed Total Fifty Six (56)	*Office use*
Signature of doctor *Nadia Bukhari*	12 May 2013 Balmoral Surgery Balmoral Road Surbiton KT5	
NHS	PATIENTS – please read the notes overleaf	

28 Assuming today's date is 4 June 2013, the above prescription cannot be dispensed because:

- ☐ A the patient's date of birth is missing
- ☐ B the prescription has expired
- ☐ C the number of days' treatment is missing
- ☐ D the pharmaceutical form of the drug is missing
- ☐ E the direction for taking the medication is missing

<table>
<tr><td>Pharmacy stamp</td><td>Age

63</td><td rowspan="2">Name (including forename) and address

R Williams

54 Scream Lane

London

W1</td></tr>
<tr><td>Number of days' treatment

N.B. Ensure dose is stated</td><td></td></tr>
<tr><td>Endorsements</td><td>Fentanyl Patch 25mcg Mdu

Total 10(ten)</td><td rowspan="3">Office use</td></tr>
<tr><td>Signature of doctor

Nadia Bukhari</td><td>15 May 2013

Balmoral Surgery

Balmoral Road

Surbiton KT5</td></tr>
<tr><td>NHS</td><td>PATIENTS – please read the notes overleaf</td></tr>
</table>

29 Assuming today's date is 4 June 2013, the above prescription cannot be dispensed because:

- ☐ A the patient's date of birth is missing
- ☐ B the prescription has expired
- ☐ C the number of days' treatment is missing
- ☐ D the pharmaceutical form of the drug is missing
- ☐ E the direction for taking the medication is not valid

<table>
<tr><td>Pharmacy stamp</td><td>Age

39</td><td rowspan="2">Name (including forename) and address

B Spears

Yule Gardens

London

W1</td></tr>
<tr><td>Number of days' treatment

N.B. Ensure dose is stated</td><td>14</td></tr>
<tr><td>Endorsements</td><td>Temazepam

Take one at night</td><td rowspan="3">Office use</td></tr>
<tr><td>Signature of doctor

Nadia Bukhari</td><td>20 May 2013

Balmoral Surgery

Balmoral Road

Surbiton KT5</td></tr>
<tr><td>NHS</td><td>PATIENTS – please read the notes overleaf</td></tr>
</table>

30 Assuming today's date is 4 June 2013, the above prescription cannot be dispensed because:

- ☐ A the prescription has expired
- ☐ B the strength of the drug is missing
- ☐ C the total quantity to dispense is missing
- ☐ D the pharmaceutical form of the drug is missing
- ☐ E the direction for taking the medication is not valid

31 Which of the following products found in the pharmacy is the least likely to be abused?

- ☐ A dextromethorphan
- ☐ B pseudoephedrine
- ☐ C glycerol
- ☐ D senna
- ☐ E phenylephrine

32 Which of the following healthcare professionals *cannot* request an emergency supply of a prescription-only medicine?

- ☐ A supplementary nurse prescriber
- ☐ B Swiss doctor
- ☐ C vet
- ☐ D dentist
- ☐ E community nurse prescriber

33 Miss XC is a regular patient of your pharmacy and comes to collect her daily instalment of methadone.
She returns, 10 minutes later, asking for another to be dispensed as she dropped the bottle containing methadone. She shows you pieces of the broken bottle. Which of the following is the most appropriate response?

- ☐ A Dispense tomorrow's methadone but contact her prescriber to obtain a prescription for next week's instalment.
- ☐ B Tell her there's nothing you can do about it.
- ☐ C Get more details about the area where she dropped it and go to have a look yourself to confirm her story. If true, supply another bottle.
- ☐ D Advise Miss XC that she must go back to her prescriber to request another prescription.
- ☐ E Inform Miss XC that you must contact the police and prescriber before dispensing any more methadone to her.

34 Digoxin is used for the treatment of heart failure. Which of the following is the correct explanation of its function? Digoxin:

- ☐ A reduces conductivity in the AV node
- ☐ B decreases the force of contraction of the heart
- ☐ C decreases blood pressure
- ☐ D increases blood pressure
- ☐ E decreases cardiac output

35 Mrs JU takes digoxin regularly. Her doctor prescribes her furosemide as she is complaining of ankle oedema. The pharmacist decides to monitor the patient regularly, as there is a potential interaction between the two drugs.
Which of the following is a correct explanation of the mechanism of the interaction?

- ☐ A Furosemide induces the metabolism of digoxin.
- ☐ B Furosemide inhibits the metabolism of digoxin.
- ☐ C Furosemide may cause hyponatraemia which predisposes to digoxin toxicity.
- ☐ D Furosemide may cause hyperkalaemia which predisposes to digoxin toxicity.
- ☐ E Furosemide given with digoxin may induce digoxin toxicity.

36 Miss TZ is taking lithium for bipolar disorder. Lithium is a drug which requires therapeutic drug monitoring. Which of the following is the correct therapeutic range for lithium?

- ☐ A 0.1–1 mmol/L
- ☐ B 0.2–2 mmol/L
- ☐ C 0.3–1 mmol/L
- ☐ D 0.4–1 mmol/L
- ☐ E 0.4–2 mmol/L

37 Miss TZ requires regular lithium monitoring. Which of the following is *not* a toxic effect of lithium poisoning?

- ☐ A ataxia
- ☐ B convulsions
- ☐ C renal failure
- ☐ D dysarthria
- ☐ E bradycardia

38 Miss TZ has come into the lithium clinic for a blood test. Which hormone requires monitoring with lithium?

- ☐ A cortisol
- ☐ B insulin
- ☐ C thyroid
- ☐ D aldosterone
- ☐ E follicle stimulating hormone

39 Which of the following interacts with lithium?

- ☐ A naproxen
- ☐ B propranolol
- ☐ C simvastatin
- ☐ D ranitidine
- ☐ E amoxicillin

40 Which of the following may be indicated for neuropathic pain?

- ☐ A ketoprofen
- ☐ B paracetamol
- ☐ C phenytoin
- ☐ D paroxetine
- ☐ E piroxicam

41 Which of the following is *not* a side effect of amitriptyline?

- ☐ A blurred vision
- ☐ B acne
- ☐ C urinary retention
- ☐ D drowsiness
- ☐ E constipation

42 Which of the following is the desired therapeutic range of phenytoin?

- ☐ A 5–10 mg/L
- ☐ B 10–20 mg/L
- ☐ C 20–30 mg/L
- ☐ D 30–40 mg/L
- ☐ E 40–50 mg/L

43 Which of the following is the correct indication for digoxin therapy?

- ☐ A hypertension
- ☐ B stable angina
- ☐ C secondary prevention post MI
- ☐ D atrial fibrillation
- ☐ E anticoagulation

44 If you have been supplied counterfeit stock, who should be contacted immediately?

- ☐ A GPhC
- ☐ B NPA
- ☐ C MHRA
- ☐ D PSNC
- ☐ E Cochrane

45 Which is false with regard to ACE inhibitor therapy?

- ☐ A it should be initiated at bedtime
- ☐ B it should be initiated with a low dose
- ☐ C it should be initiated in the community
- ☐ D it may cause a dry cough
- ☐ E ACE inhibitors may decrease the excretion of certain drugs

46 Which of the following drugs causes significant gastro-intestinal disturbance which requires slow upward titration of its dosing regimen?

- ☐ A metformin
- ☐ B atenolol
- ☐ C prednisolone
- ☐ D lisinopril
- ☐ E levothyroxine

47 Ms DL is admitted on your ward. She is on a heparin infusion and has received a higher than normal dose. You urgently bleep the SHO to prescribe a drug to reverse heparin. Which of the following do you recommend?

- ☐ A vitamin K
- ☐ B protamine
- ☐ C naloxone
- ☐ D charcoal
- ☐ E stomach lavage

48 Mr HF is taking pioglitazone for type 2 diabetes mellitus. Which of the following requires immediate medical attention when taking this drug?

- ☐ A liver toxicity
- ☐ B renal impairment
- ☐ C sore throat
- ☐ D GI disturbance
- ☐ E weight loss

49 Which of the following drugs may cause a sudden onset of sleep?

- ☐ A omeprazole
- ☐ B adrenaline
- ☐ C pyrazinamide
- ☐ D levodopa
- ☐ E ondansetron

50 Which of the following is *not* a risk factor for venous thromboembolism in patients taking the oral contraceptive?

- ☐ A age over 35 years
- ☐ B obesity
- ☐ C family history
- ☐ D smoking
- ☐ E hypertension

MULTIPLE COMPLETION QUESTIONS

Each of the questions or incomplete statements in this section is followed by three responses.

For each question, ONE or MORE of the responses is/are correct. Decide which of the responses is/are correct, then choose:

A if 1, 2 and 3 are correct
B if 1 and 2 only are correct
C if 2 and 3 only are correct
D if 1 only is correct
E if 3 only is correct

Summary				
A	B	C	D	E
1, 2, 3	1, 2 only	2, 3 only	1 only	3 only

1 Regarding enzyme inducers and inhibitors, which of the following is/are true?

- ☐ 1 Phenobarbital is an enzyme inducer.
- ☐ 2 Enzyme induction may take up to 2–3 weeks to wear off.
- ☐ 3 Enzyme inhibition takes 4 weeks to wear off.

2 Regarding the NHS recommendations for alcohol consumption, which of the following is/are true?

- ☐ 1 For men, the alcohol limit is 3–4 units per day.
- ☐ 2 For women, the alcohol limit is 2–3 units per day.
- ☐ 3 If a person has had a heavy drinking session, he/she should avoid alcohol for 48 hours.

3 The use of some drugs in patients with renal impairment can have which of the following effect(s)?

- ☐ 1 reduced sensitivity to some drugs including cases where drug elimination is unaffected
- ☐ 2 poor tolerance to drug side-effects
- ☐ 3 few or no therapeutic effects

4 Which of the following statements is/are true regarding ciprofloxacin?

- ☐ 1 It is an inhibitor of CYP450.
- ☐ 2 It can reduce the seizure threshold and is therefore contraindicated in patients with a history of a seizure, including epilepsy.
- ☐ 3 It is contraindicated in children under the age of 12.

5 Regarding the use of hormone replacement therapy (HRT), which of the following statements is/are true?

- ☐ 1 HRT can be used as a contraceptive.
- ☐ 2 Oestrogen increases the risk of postmenopausal osteoporosis.
- ☐ 3 HRT must be stopped immediately if the patient experiences severe stomach pain.

6 You wish to take a thorough medication history. Which of the following sources can be used?

- ☐ 1 patient medical record
- ☐ 2 hospital discharge summaries
- ☐ 3 patient or their representatives

7 Which of the following antibiotics can cause *Clostridium difficile* infection?

- ☐ 1 vancomycin
- ☐ 2 clindamycin
- ☐ 3 ciprofloxacin

8 The following are prescription extracts. For which of these extracts would you need to contact the prescriber to obtain further details before dispensing the medication?

- ☐ 1 'hypromellose eye drops'
- ☐ 2 'theophylline m/r tablets'
- ☐ 3 'nifidipine m/r tablets'

9 Which of the following statements is/are true regarding continuing professional development (CPD)?

- ☐ 1 Registered pharmacists must complete a minimum of 12 CPD entries per registered year.
- ☐ 2 All entries must include all of the CPD cycle stages as outlined by the General Pharmaceutical Council (GPhC).
- ☐ 3 Learning from *The Pharmaceutical Journal* can be considered as CPD activity.

10 Which of the following statements is/are true with regard to the propionic acid derivative ibuprofen?

- ☐ 1 Ibuprofen has anti-inflammatory, analgesic and antipyretic properties.
- ☐ 2 In adults, the maximum daily dose is 2.4 g (in divided doses).
- ☐ 3 It has the least incidence of side-effects compared with other non-selective NSAIDS.

11 Which of the following drugs is/are unsuitable for use in children?

- ☐ 1 guaifenesin
- ☐ 2 dextromethorphan
- ☐ 3 chlorphenamine

12 Regarding expiry dates and medicines for disposal, which of the following statements is/are true?

- ☐ 1 Pharmacies can receive waste medicines.
- ☐ 2 A product with an expiry date of 12/2013 should not be used after 31/12/2013.
- ☐ 3 'Use by 12/2013' means that the product should not be used after 31/12/2013.

13 Which of the following substances has/have anxiogenic effects?

☐ 1 caffeine
☐ 2 levodopa
☐ 3 diazepam

14 Which of the following can cause acute urticaria?

☐ 1 latex
☐ 2 shellfish
☐ 3 ibuprofen

15 Your manager asks you to give a seminar on drugs with a narrow therapeutic index. Which of the following drugs can you select for your presentation?

☐ 1 phenytoin
☐ 2 minoxidil
☐ 3 carbamazepine

16 Which of the following preparations may be used to ease the symptoms associated with scabies?

☐ 1 calamine lotion
☐ 2 crotamiton
☐ 3 short-term use of chlorphenamine

17 Which of the following pathogenic organisms lead to infections which have been transmitted via the faecal-oral route?

☐ 1 *Escherichia coli*
☐ 2 *Shigella dysenteriae*
☐ 3 *Vibrio cholerae*

18 To avoid any errors in dispensing, which of the following words should not be abbreviated on prescriptions?

☐ 1 micrograms
☐ 2 units
☐ 3 nanograms

19 Which of the following stain(s) teeth?

- ☐ 1 hexetidine mouthwash
- ☐ 2 chlorhexidine gluconate mouthwash
- ☐ 3 doxycycline capsules

20 Which of the following parasites are species of round worm?

- ☐ 1 hookworm
- ☐ 2 pinworm
- ☐ 3 whipworm

21 Dr N, the FY1 on your ward, is discussing a patient case with you. She points out that one of the patients has been wrongly diagnosed with cancer. Which of the following conditions is/are not a type of cancer?

- ☐ 1 granuloma
- ☐ 2 cerebral astrocytoma
- ☐ 3 Ewing's sarcoma

22 Which of the following substances is/are available in all three legal groups: GSL, P and POM?

- ☐ 1 aspirin
- ☐ 2 clotrimazole
- ☐ 3 chlorphenamine

23 Which of the following infections may be contracted by airborne transmission?

- ☐ 1 anthrax
- ☐ 2 smallpox
- ☐ 3 meningitis

24 Mr A wishes to purchase *Peptac* from your pharmacy. According to your knowledge of physiology, you should advise Mr A not to take *Peptac* 2 hours before or after which of the following medicines?

- ☐ 1 sulfasalazine e/c
- ☐ 2 ketoconazole
- ☐ 3 minocycline

25 Which of the following terminologies can be used interchangeably with a disease that is 'cryptogenic'?

☐ 1 idiopathic
☐ 2 asymptomatic
☐ 3 chronic

26 Which of the following is/are non-communicable diseases?

☐ 1 chronic obstructive pulmonary disease
☐ 2 diabetes mellitus
☐ 3 cardiovascular disease

27 Which of the following is/are used in the management of opioid dependence and withdrawal symptoms?

☐ 1 methadone
☐ 2 lofexidine
☐ 3 loperamide

28 Which of the following substances is/are available as GSL only?

☐ 1 mepyramine maleate
☐ 2 colecalciferol
☐ 3 dimeticone

29 Which of the following is/are considered localised diseases?

☐ 1 gout
☐ 2 cluster headache
☐ 3 multiple sclerosis

30 You are asked to give a seminar to the hospital staff on eating disorders. Which of the following is/are types of eating disorders?

☐ 1 anorexia nervosa
☐ 2 bulimia nervosa
☐ 3 pica

31 A woman comes into your pharmacy asking for the 'morning after pill'. She had unprotected sex eight hours ago and is not taking any medications. Given that there are no contraindications, which of the following is/are suitable?

- ☐ 1 levonorgestrel 1.5 mg tablet
- ☐ 2 intra-uterine device
- ☐ 3 *FemSeven* Conti

32 Which of the following cancers are often caused by asbestos exposure?

- ☐ 1 melanoma
- ☐ 2 non-Hodgkin's lymphoma
- ☐ 3 mesothelioma

33 With regards to nicotine replacement therapy (NRT) which of the following statements is/are true?

- ☐ 1 All NRT preparations are licensed for adults and children over 12.
- ☐ 2 Nicotine is present in breast milk.
- ☐ 3 NRT should be used with caution in patients with diabetes mellitus.

34 Drug misusers are susceptible to contracting blood-borne viruses. Regarding this, which of the following statements is/are true?

- ☐ 1 Hepatitis A is commonly transmitted through the oral-faecal route.
- ☐ 2 Hepatitis B and C, and HIV are transmitted via sexual intercourse.
- ☐ 3 Vaccination is currently available against hepatitis A and B viruses but not against hepatitis C.

35 Which of the following is/are used in the management of alcohol dependence?

- ☐ 1 naltrexone
- ☐ 2 disulfiram
- ☐ 3 thiamine

36 Which of the following is a non-sedating antihistamine which is licensed for the symptomatic relief of seasonal allergic rhinitis in an 8-year-old child (given no other contraindications)?

- ☐ **1** fexofenadine
- ☐ **2** acrivastine
- ☐ **3** promethazine

37 Miss K, a 29-year-old female, is talking to you about her summer plans while you are preparing her medications. She tells you that she is getting a fake tan and has already 'booked a sunbed' for later this week. You should warn Miss K not to use sunbeds if she is taking:

- ☐ **1** isotretinoin
- ☐ **2** amiodarone
- ☐ **3** co-trimoxazole

38 Which of the following is/are a preparation of epinephrine?

- ☐ **1** *Epipen*
- ☐ **2** *Jext*
- ☐ **3** *Cinryze*

39 Which of the following conditions is/are genetically inherited?

- ☐ **1** beta-thalassaemia
- ☐ **2** haemophilia
- ☐ **3** Turner syndrome

40 Which of the following conditions can affect the vulvovaginal region of the body?

- ☐ **1** vaginitis
- ☐ **2** candida albicans
- ☐ **3** trichomoniasis

41 Which of the following is/are associated with a localised demarcated plaque?

- ☐ **1** lichen simplex
- ☐ **2** psoriasis
- ☐ **3** *Listeria monocytogenes*

42 Which of the following statements relate(s) to ciprofloxacin?

☐ **1** It reduces the seizure threshold and is therefore cautioned in epilepsy.
☐ **2** It is an CYP3A4 inhibitor.
☐ **3** It is contraindicated in children under the age of 12.

43 Which of the following drugs have a short-duration of action?

☐ **1** glyceryl trinitrate
☐ **2** terbutaline
☐ **3** atorvastatin

44 Hypersensivity reactions have been associated with which of the following drugs?

☐ **1** lisinopril
☐ **2** naproxen
☐ **3** balsalazide

45 Which of the following statements is/are true regarding 5HT1-receptor agonists?

☐ **1** Zolmitriptan is an example of a 5HT1-receptor agonist.
☐ **2** They are used in the treatment of migraine.
☐ **3** They should not be used in patients who have had a heart attack.

46 Mr K comes into your pharmacy complaining of 'stomach pain'. In which of the following situations would you need to refer him to his GP?

☐ **1** if he reports haematemesis
☐ **2** sudden weight loss
☐ **3** halitosis

47 Mrs Z is a 32-year-old pregnant woman who is 28 weeks pregnant. She comes into your pharmacy asking for some OTC medications for herself. Which of the following products is/are not suitable for her?

☐ **1** *Pepto Bismol*
☐ **2** *Sudafed*
☐ **3** *Galcodine*

48 Mr K, a regular customer in your pharmacy, asks you about a recent article he has read in a magazine about herbal products. Which of the following statements is/are true?

- ☐ 1 Black cohosh may cause rare but serious liver toxicity.
- ☐ 2 Gingko biloba can interfere with the action of anaesthetics.
- ☐ 3 Some herbal medicines contain heavy metals such as arsenic sulphide.

49 For which of the following substances has the number of pack sizes available under GSL classification increased?

- ☐ 1 hyoscine butylbromide
- ☐ 2 loratadine
- ☐ 3 loperamide

50 Which of the following ectoparasites live on hair follicles?

- ☐ 1 *Sarcoptes scabiei*
- ☐ 2 *Phthirus pubis*
- ☐ 3 *Pediculus humanus*

51 You are the pharmacist on duty in the hospital in-patient dispensary. You receive a prescription for busulfan. Which of the following statements is/are true?

- ☐ 1 Busulfan is a cytotoxic agent.
- ☐ 2 Protective clothing (such as gloves, gowns and masks) should be worn when handling any cytotoxic agent.
- ☐ 3 Irreversible hair loss is a common side-effect of cytotoxic agents.

52 You are a locum pharmacist who has been called to cover a shift at a pharmacy in a walk-in centre. It is your responsibility to ensure that a notice, indicating that you are responsible for the safe and effective running of the registered pharmacy, is clearly displayed to the public. What information must be displayed on the notice?

- ☐ 1 your full name
- ☐ 2 your registration number
- ☐ 3 that you are the responsible pharmacist who is currently in charge of the pharmacy premises

53 Mr A is a 42-year-old male who has recently been admitted to your ward for unexplained seizures and blurred vision. He has a BMI of 26 kg/m^2 and his recent blood results show a HbA_{1c} of 65 mmol/mol. Which of the following statements is/are true?

- ☐ 1 Mr A is likely to be suffering from diabetes mellitus.
- ☐ 2 Where there are no other influential factors on the measurement of HbA_{1c}, a value of 48 mmol/mol (6.5%) is the recommended cut point for the diagnosis of diabetes mellitus.
- ☐ 3 Anaemia can interfere with HbA_{1c} measurements.

54 The Misuse of Drugs Act classifies illicit drugs into three categories: A, B or C. Regarding this, which of the following statements is/are true?

- ☐ 1 Class A drugs pose the most risk to health, whereas class C drugs pose the least risk.
- ☐ 2 Amfetamines are powerful stimulants which are also known by the name ‘speed’.
- ☐ 3 Cannabis and cocaine are examples of class A drugs.

55 Mrs K is a 28-year-old female who comes into your pharmacy complaining of dyspepsia. Which of the following requires urgent medical referral?

- ☐ 1 upper abdominal pain
- ☐ 2 haematemesis
- ☐ 3 weight loss

56 You are the responsible pharmacist at a community pharmacy who is carrying out a controlled drug (CD) stock count. While checking the CD register you notice *all* of the drugs inside the CD cabinet have been included in the register. Which of the following CDs do not require recording in the CD register?

- ☐ 1 quinalbarbitone
- ☐ 2 phenobarbital
- ☐ 3 midazolam

57 Which of the following statements is/are true regarding the duration of action of drugs?

☐ 1 Insulin detemir is a short-acting human insulin analogue.
☐ 2 Terbutaline inhaler, glyceryl trinitrate sublingual tablets and zopiclone tablets are all short-acting preparations.
☐ 3 Phenobarbital and salmeterol are both long-acting preparations.

58 Mrs P is a 29-year-old female who has just returned from Assam in India. She tells you that she has been feeling very poorly and describes her symptoms to you. Which of the following symptoms may indicate that Mrs P could have contracted malaria?

☐ 1 myalgia
☐ 2 flu-like symptoms such as fever, sweats and chills
☐ 3 red spots which do not blanch with pressure

59 Which of the following statements is/are correct with regard to extemporaneously prepared formulations?

☐ 1 Freshly prepared preparations must be made within 48 hours from date of issue.
☐ 2 Recently prepared preparations should be used within 4 weeks from date of preparation.
☐ 3 Potable water is water which is drawn from the public supply and is suitable for drinking.

60 Mr K is the responsible pharmacist who is working with you on the outpatient ward. At 1 pm Mr K asks you to cover his absence between 2.30 and 5 pm as he needs to pick up his daughter from school. There are no other pharmacists available to cover his shift during this period. Which of the following responses is/are correct?

☐ 1 Tell Mr K to remove the responsible pharmacist notice from display during his absence.
☐ 2 Tell Mr K that you can cover his absence, as you can take your lunch later in the afternoon.
☐ 3 Ask Mr K to make arrangements as neither of you can leave for a period which exceeds two hours.

61 All solid, oral and external liquid preparations must be dispensed in child-resistant containers at all times with exceptions in certain situations. In which of the following scenarios would an exception apply?

- ☐ 1 a 73-year-old patient with arthritic hands
- ☐ 2 you receive a prescription for *Incivo* tablets which contain a desiccant in their original package
- ☐ 3 the pharmacy dispensary has run out of child-resistant bottles

62 Which of the following statements is/are true with regard to pharmacy-related sources?

- ☐ 1 The National Institute for Health and Care Excellence (NICE), the Scottish Medicines Consortium (SMC) and the Scottish Intercollegiate Guidelines Network (SIGN) all produce consensus guidelines.
- ☐ 2 The NHS Business Service Authority provides information for prices of medicinal products and appliances.
- ☐ 3 Summaries of Product information (SPCs) are documents containing detailed information regarding a medication's dosage, pharmacokinetics and storage.

CLASSIFICATION QUESTIONS

In this section, for each numbered question, select the one lettered option that most closely corresponds to the answer. Within each group of questions each lettered option may be used once, more than once or not at all.

Questions 1–4 concern the following drugs:

- A lithium
- B warfarin
- C metronidazole
- D prednisolone (long-term use)
- E moclobemide

For each of the statements below select the drug to which it applies.

1 This drug is not issued with a warning card.
2 Patients taking this should avoid alcohol for at least 1 week after stopping treatment.
3 Patients taking this should avoid excessive consumption of mature cheese.
4 A patient taking this may present with memory loss.

Questions 5–7 concern the following ingredients:

- A calamine
- B acacia
- C liquid paraffin
- D phenol liquid
- E zinc oxide

Which of the above ingredients:

5 burns the skin?
6 may be used as an active ingredient in barrier preparations?
7 is present in preparations which can be used for the treatment of dry eyes?

Questions 8–9 concern the following conditions:

- A dehydration
- B fever
- C pancreatitis
- D septic shock
- E hypoalbuminaemia

For each of the following statements, select the condition that is being described.

8 Dry mouth, lips and eyes, dark urine and lethargy are signs of this clinical state.
9 Is a common side-effect which may follow a vaccine injection.

Questions 10–13 concern the following commonly used medical abbreviations:

- A SOB
- B MI
- C TPN
- D CVA
- E LMP

Select from A to E, which of the above corresponds to:

10 a heart attack
11 dyspnoea
12 stroke
13 the last date of a patient's menstrual period

Questions 14–17 concern the following ocular conditions:

- A dry eyes
- B wet age-related macular degeneration
- C primary open angle glaucoma
- D amblyopia
- E hypermetropia

Select from A to E, which of the above corresponds to:

14 a condition where the production of abnormal, leaky blood vessels leads to central vision loss
15 can be caused by meibomian glands dysfunction
16 topical beta-blockers can be used to treat this condition
17 is the term used to describe farsighted people

Questions 18–21 concern the following actions:

A Advise the patient to discontinue the treatment and seek medical attention immediately.
B Advise the patient to see their GP as a dose adjustment or a change of medication may be necessary.
C Advise the patient to seek immediate medical attention.
D Advise the patient that the reported side-effect is commonly associated with their medication. They may choose to continue with the treatment or ask their GP for an alternative.
E Advise the patient that the described sign is not commonly associated with their treatment.

Select from A to E, which of the above actions is correct for the following scenarios:

18 a patient taking insulin detemir who complains of perspiration and feeling hungry
19 a patient taking phenytoin who complains of a mouth ulcer and feeling 'feverish'
20 a patient taking levothyroxine who complains of chronic constipation
21 a patient taking warfarin who complains of constipation

Questions 22–25 concern the following skin conditions:

A warts
B psoriasis
C vitiligo
D ringworm
E impetigo

Select from A to E, which of the following signs correspond to the above conditions:

22 skin rash with an appearance of an inflamed ring with a healing centre
23 a raised lesion with a cauliflower appearance
24 dry, red lesions covered with silver scales
25 white patches of skin which are the result of little or no melanin production

Questions 26–28 concern the following drugs:

A furosemide
B indapamide
C citalopram
D moclobemide
E sevelamer

Select from A to E, which of the above drugs:

26 acts on the distal convoluted tubule
27 is a monoamine reuptake inhibitor
28 binds to phosphate

Questions 29–32 concern the following therapeutic agents:

A infliximab
B tranexamic acid
C amiodarone
D zolmitriptan
E peppermint oil

Select from A to E, which of the above belong to the following classes of drugs:

29 TNF-α inhibitor
30 antiarrhythmic agent
31 antifibrinolytic agent
32 antispasmodic agent

Questions 33–35 concern the following drug overdoses:

- A aspirin
- B paracetamol
- C pethidine
- D iron
- E epinephrine

Select from A to E, for which drugs the following substances are used in the management of drug poisoning:

33 acetylcysteine
34 desferrioxamine
35 naloxone

Questions 36–39 concern the following foot conditions:

- A corn
- B bunion
- C blister
- D gout
- E chilblain

Select from A to E, the condition which is described below:

36 a bony swelling at the base of the big toe
37 a pocket of fluid which appears in the upper layer of the skin
38 a small, itchy swelling on the skin which results from cold temperature
39 a painful swelling in the joints as a result of uric acid build up in the blood

Questions 40–43 concern the following conditions:

- A chickenpox
- B measles
- C head lice
- D mumps
- E scabies

Select from A to E, which of the above corresponds to:

40 red-brown rash which starts behind the ears and spreads around the head and neck then to the rest of the body
41 wingless insects which live by sucking blood and laying white eggs also known as nits
42 starts as a small itchy rash which develops into blisters
43 parasites which burrow into the skin

Questions 44–47 concern the following vitamins:

A folic acid
B vitamin A
C vitamin D
D vitamin K
E vitamin B_6

Select from A to E, which of the above vitamins correspond to the following statements:

44 deficiency of this vitamin may occur with isoniazid therapy
45 when taken before and during pregnancy, this supplement reduces the risk of developing fetal spina bifida
46 is teratogenic
47 is given as a supplement to neonates to prevent bleeding

Questions 48–51 concern the classes of vitamin B:

A vitamin B_1
B vitamin B_2
C vitamin B_6
D vitamin B_{12}
E vitamin B_3

Select from A to E, which of the above corresponds to:

48 is also known as riboflavin
49 patients with pernicious anaemia are deficient in this vitamin
50 prolonged use of high doses of this vitamin has been associated with peripheral nerve damage
51 use of the amide form (nicotinamide) of this vitamin is preferred as it does not cause vasodilatation

Questions 52–55 concern the following respiratory tract signs:

A tachypnoea
B bradypnoea
C dyspnoea
D hypoxia
E haemoptysis

Select from A to E, which of the above corresponds to:

52 slow rate of breathing
53 rapid rate of breathing
54 shortness of breath
55 coughing out blood

Questions 56–59 concern the following signs:

A haematochezia
B haemoptysis
C haemangioma
D hemiballismus
E haematuria

Select from A to E, which one of the above signs presents as:

56 vascular birthmarks on the skin which are often called 'strawberry marks'
57 blood from the respiratory tract following a cough
58 violent, involuntary flinging motions of the extremities
59 fresh red blood in stools

Questions 60–63 concern the following Latin abbreviations:

A gtt.
B p.c.
C o.u.
D Sig.
E p.r.

Select from A to E, which one of the above Latin abbreviations stands for:

60 drops
61 both eyes
62 after food
63 rectally

Questions 64–67 concern the following gastro-intestinal signs and symptoms:

A melaena
B odynophagia
C dysphagia
D steatorrhoea
E pyrosis

Select from A to E, which of the above corresponds to:

64 painful swallowing
65 fatty stools
66 tarry stools
67 heartburn

Questions 68–71 concern the following proprietary preparations:

A *Nitrolingual Pumpspray*
B *Asasantin Retard* capsules
C *Zocor* tablets
D *Fosamax* tablets
E *Ovestin*

Select from A to E, which of the above corresponds to:

68 preparation should be dispensed in original container and discarded 6 weeks after opening
69 is available as a P medication containing simvastatin 10 mg tablets
70 is a sublingual preparation which can be used to provide rapid symptomatic relief of angina
71 contains alendronic acid

Questions 72–75 concern the following neurological signs and symptoms:

A anomic aphasia
B allochiria
C dysarthria
D ataxia
E dystonia

Select from A to E, in which of the above situations a person would:

72 have difficulties in recalling names or words
73 have difficulties in coordinating voluntary muscle movements
74 perceive stimuli in the opposite side of the body
75 have difficulties in speech articulation

Questions 76–79 concern the following brands:

A *Tritace*
B *Xenical*
C *Atrovent*
D *Zyprexa*
E *Tegretol*

Select from A to E, the suitable preparations which can be indicated in the following conditions:

76 asthma
77 hypertension
78 schizophrenia
79 epilepsy

STATEMENT QUESTIONS

The questions in this section consist of a statement in the top row followed by a second statement beneath.

You need to:

decide whether the *first statement* is true or false

decide whether the *second statement* is true or false

Then choose:

- A if both statements are true and the second statement is *a correct explanation* of the first statement
- B if both statements are true but the second statement is *not a correct explanation* of the first statement
- C if the first statement is true but the second statement is false
- D if the first statement is false but the second statement is true
- E if both statements are false

1 **First statement**

CPD entries can start at the planning phase of the cycle

Second statement

Evaluation comes at the end of the CPD cycle

2 **First statement**

The age of the patient must be stated on an FP10 form

Second statement

Having the age on the prescription for patients who are under 16 years of age is a legal requirement

3 **First statement**

Repeatable prescriptions can be issued on FP10 forms

Second statement

If there is no quantity of the repeat stated, then they cannot be repeated

4 **First statement**

Dentists can write prescriptions legally for any POM

Second statement

When prescribing on an NHS dental form, they can only prescribe medicines listed in the *Dental Practitioners' Formulary*

5 **First statement**

Doctors registered in an EEA country can order emergency supplies from a pharmacist in the UK

Second statement

Countries in the EEA include Italy, Malta and Turkey

6 **First statement**

Dentists registered in the UK can request an emergency supply for a patient

Second statement

The original prescription *must* be obtained within 24 hours

7 **First statement**

Pharmacists can be connected to ex-directory numbers in an emergency

Second statement

A pharmacist needing to contact an ex-directory number should dial 101

8 **First statement**

The name of the animal *must* be written on a veterinary prescription

Second statement

'As directed' is not accepted as an administration instruction on veterinary prescriptions

9 **First statement**

Schedule 3 controlled drugs are exempt from controlled drug prescription requirements

Second statement

Schedule 3 controlled drugs prescriptions are valid for 6 months

10 **First statement**

Controlled drugs requisitions must have the purpose of the requisition stated on it

Second statement

Standard requisition forms have been introduced since the Shipman Inquiry

11 **First statement**

Potassium levels should be monitored with digoxin therapy

Second statement

Digoxin causes hypokalaemia as a side-effect

12 **First statement**

Patients on amiodarone therapy should avoid exposure to sunlight

Second statement

Amiodarone therapy causes corneal micro deposits in the eye causing night glare

13 **First statement**

Beta-blockers can be used in heart failure

Second statement

Bisoprolol is a beta-blocker

14 **First statement**

NSAIDs should not be given at the same time as ciprofloxacin

Second statement

NSAIDs reduce the excretion of ciprofloxacin, causing seizures

15 **First statement**

H. pylori eradication usually involves triple therapy

Second statement

Triple therapy consists of a PPI, an H2 receptor antagonist with a suitable antibiotic

16 **First statement**

Nicorandil is licensed for the treatment of stable angina

Second statement

Nicorandil is a vasodilator

17 **First statement**

ACE inhibitors are recommended to be initiated at night

Second statement

ACE inhibitors may cause drowsiness

18 **First statement**

If a patient complains of tendon pain while on ciprofloxacin therapy, the drug should be discontinued

Second statement

Ciprofloxacin can cause tendon damage

19 **First statement**

Convulsions may occur in patients taking long-term fluoxetine therapy

Second statement

Fluoxetine may cause hyponatraemia

20 **First statement**

Salmeterol is a long-acting beta-2 agonist

Second statement

Salmeterol can be introduced in step 1 in the management of chronic asthma

21 **First statement**

Clozapine is indicated for bipolar disorder

Second statement

Agranulocytosis is associated with clozapine therapy

22 **First statement**

Broad bean pods should be avoided while taking phenelzine

Second statement

The interaction between monoamine oxidase inhibitors and tyramine can cause a dangerous rise in blood pressure

23 **First statement**

Flucloxacillin should not be used in patients with hepatic dysfunction

Second statement

Flucloxacillin may cause cholestatic jaundice

24 **First statement**

Clindamycin is associated with fatal colitis

Second statement

Clindamycin can be used to treat cellulitis

25 **First statement**

Metformin causes hypoglycaemia as a side-effect

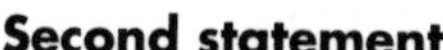

Second statement

There is an increased risk of lactic acidosis in patients with renal impairment taking metformin therapy

26 **First statement**

Hypertension is a side-effect of prednisolone therapy

Second statement

Hypertension is a mineralocorticoid side-effect

27 **First statement**

Finasteride is indicated for benign prostatic hyperplasia

Second statement

Women of child-bearing potential should avoid handling crushed or broken tablets of finasteride

28 **First statement**

Dry mouth is a side-effect of procyclidine

Second statement

Procyclidine is an antimuscarinic drug

29 **First statement**

Patients on lithium therapy should maintain adequate salt intake

Second statement

Lithium may cause hypernatraemia

30 **First statement**

When initiating metformin in a patient, the dose should be gradually titrated to the desired dosing regime

Second statement

Metformin may cause severe gastro-intestinal disturbances

31 **First statement**

Alendronic acid should be taken with a full glass of water

Second statement

Alendronic acid may cause severe oesophageal reactions

32 **First statement**

Diamorphine is a schedule 1 controlled drug

Second statement

Naloxone can be used to reverse respiratory depression with opioids

33 **First statement**

Propranolol should not be given with pseudoephedrine

Second statement

Antihypertensives and sympathomimetics can cause severe hypotension when given together

34 **First statement**

Hydrocortisone cream 1% should not be sold over the counter to children under 12 years

Second statement

Hydrocortisone 1% cream should be applied thinly

35 **First statement**

Warfarin is a narrow therapeutic drug

Second statement

Warfarin may cause haemorrhage as a side-effect

36 **First statement**

Amiodarone and atenolol should not be used concurrently

Second statement

Amiodarone and beta-blockers may cause heart block when given together

37 **First statement**

Furosemide may precipitate gout

Second statement

Furosemide causes hypomagnesaemia

38 **First statement**

Loratadine may be prescribed for allergic rhinitis

Second statement

Loratadine may cause blurred vision

39 **First statement**

Lorazepam can be indicated for long-term use in anxiety

Second statement

Patients taking lorazepam should be warned not to drive or perform skilled tasks

40 **First statement**

Metoclopramide is used in adults for nausea

Second statement

Metoclopramide should be used with caution in an 18-year-old girl as it is more likely to cause extrapyramidal effects

Open book answers

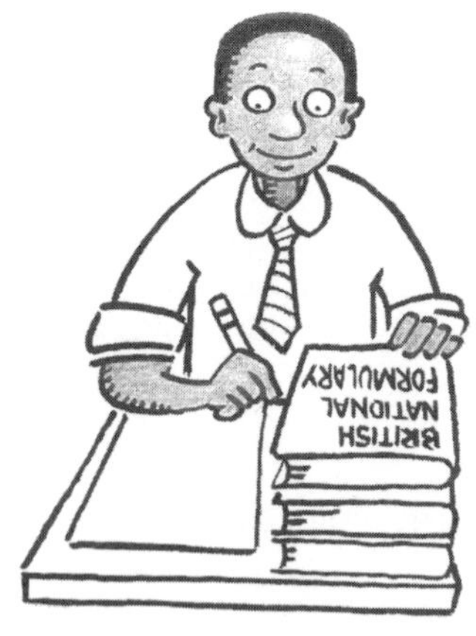

SIMPLE COMPLETION ANSWERS

1 E
See BNF, Chapter 5 (Infections), section 5.1, Antibacterial drugs, Table 1. Summary of antibacterial therapy, pyelonephritis: acute

2 D
See BNF, Chapter 9 (Nutrition and blood), section 9.5.2.2, Phosphate-binding agents, Calcium salts

3 B
See BNF, Chapter 15 (Anaesthesia), section 15.1.5, Neuromuscular blocking drugs, Non-depolarising neuromuscular blocking drugs, vecuronium bromide

4 C
Long-term use of azithromycin can cause reversible hearing loss with tinnitus. See BNF, Chapter 5 (Infections), section 5.1.5, Macrolides, side-effects

5 D
See BNF, Chapter 2 (Cardiovascular system), section 2.5.5.3, Renin inhibitors, aliskiren

6 E
See BNF, Chapter 2 (Cardiovascular system), section 2.6.4, Peripheral vasodilators and related drugs, renal impairment

7 C
See BNF, Chapter 5 (Infections), section 5.1, Antibacterial drugs, Table 2. Summary of antibacterial prophylaxis, Prevention of tuberculosis in susceptible close contacts or those who have become tuberculin positive

8 B
See BNF, Chapter 2 (Cardiovascular system), section 2.11, Antifibrinolytic drugs and haemostatics, Tranexamic acid

9 C
Disulfiram causes halitosis which is the state of having foul-smelling breath. See BNF, Chapter 4 (Central nervous system), section 4.10.1, Alcohol dependence

10 D
See BNF, Chapter 5 (Infections), section 5.3.2.1, Herpes simplex and varicella-zoster infection, famciclovir

11 D
See BNF, Chapter 6 (Endocrine system), section 6.1 Drugs used in diabetes, Measurement of HbA1c, Equivalent values

12 C
Heterochromia iridis is a condition in which a person has differently coloured irises. Prostaglandin analogues can cause darkening of the iris. See BNF, Chapter 11 (Eye), section 11.6 Treatment of glaucoma, Prostaglandin analogues and prostamides

13 D
See BNF, Chapter 5 (Infections), section 5.1.1.3, Broad-spectrum penicillins, co-amoxiclav

14 E
See BNF, Chapter 2 (Cardiovascular system), section 2.4, Beta-adrenoceptor blocking drugs, bisoprolol

15 C
See BNF, Chapter 5 (Infections), section 5.1.1.4, Antipseudomonal penicillins, Ticarcillin with clavulanic acid

16 D
See BNF, Chapter 5 (Infections), section 5.1.1.3, Broad-spectrum penicillins, amoxicillin

17 C
See BNF, Chapter 4 (Central nervous system), section 4.1.1, Hypnotics, Benzodiazepines, flurazepam

18 D
See BNF, Appendix 1 (Interactions), List of drug interactions, Angiotensin-II Receptor Antagonists, candesartan

19 D
See BNF, Chapter 1 (Gastro-intestinal system), section 1.3.1, H2-receptor antagonists, cimetidine

20 B
See BNF, Chapter 3 (Respiratory system), section 3.1.3, Theophylline, theophylline, Modified release

21 D
See BNF, Chapter 6 (Endocrine system), section 6.1.6, Diagnostic and monitoring devices for diabetes mellitus, Blood monitoring, meters and test strips

22 E
See BNF, Appendix 3 (Cautionary and advisory labels for dispensed medicines), Product Label List

23 E
See BNF, Chapter 13 (Skin), section 13.4, Topical corticosteroids, Fluticasone propionate

24 E
See BNF, Chapter 14 (Immunological products and vaccines), section 14.1, Active immunity, Immunisation schedule

25 D
See BNF, Appendix 2 (Borderline substances), section A2.4.1.1, High-energy supplements: carbohydrate, *Polycal*

26 B
See BNF, Appendix 3 (Cautionary and advisory labels for dispensed medicines), Product Label List

27 D
The use of isotretinoin has been associated with granulomatous lesions. See BNF, Chapter 13 (Skin), section 13.6.2, Oral preparations for acne, Oral retinoid for acne, isotretinoin; Armstrong, K. and Weinstein, M. (2011) Pyogenic granulomas during isotretinoin therapy. *J. Dermatol. Case Rep*. 5(1): 5–7; Teknetzis, A., Ioannides, D., Vakali, G., Lefaki, I. and Minas, A. (2004) Pyogenic granulomas following topical application of tretinoin. *J. Eur. Acad. Dermatol. Venereol*. 18(3): 337–9.

28 E
Hypertrichosis is the medical term for excessive body hair which has been reported with topical use of corticosteroids and can be avoided by applying thinly to the affected region(s) only. See BNF, Chapter 13 (Skin), section 13.4, Topical corticosteroids

29 B
When preparing potassium chloride infusions it is vital to mix the preparation very well to avoid 'layering' as this will have adverse effects on the heart if administered to the patient. See BNF, Appendix 4 (Intravenous additives), Method, potassium chloride

30 E
See BNF, Chapter 5 (Infections), section 5.1, Table 2. Summary of antibacterial prophylaxis, Prevention of infection from animal and human bites

31 D
See BNF, Dental Practitioners' Formulary, List of Dental Preparations

32 C
Diplopia means double vision. See BNF, Chapter 4 (Central nervous system), section 4.1.1, Hypnotics, Zaleplon, zolpidem, and zopiclone, Zolpidem tartrate

33 D
See BNF, Chapter 4 (Central nervous system), section 4.2.2, Antipsychotic depot injections, Equivalent doses of depot antipsychotics

34 C
Nitrates are potent coronary vasodilators and are commonly associated with postural hypotension, flushing and headache. See BNF, Chapter 2 (Cardiovascular system), section 2.6.1, Nitrates

35 D
See BNF, Chapter 5 (Infections), section 5.1.12, Quinolones, contraindications

36 B
See BNF, Chapter 10 (Musculoskeletal and joint diseases), section 10.3.2, Rubefacients, topical NSAIDs, capsaicin and poultices

37 D
Tramadol is an opioid analgesic which can also enhance serotonergic (and adrenergic) pathways. See BNF, Chapter 4 (Central nervous system), section 4.7.2, Opioid analgesics, Tramadol hydrochloride

38 E
See BNF, Chapter 5 (Infections), section 5.1.5, Macrolides

39 D
See BNF, individual drug monographs under 'renal impairment'.

40 E
See BNF, Chapter 3 (Respiratory system), section 3.9.2, Demulcent and expectorant cough preparations

41 C
See BNF, Chapter 1 (Gastro-intestinal system), section 1.6.2, Stimulant laxatives, Danthron

42 D
See BNF, Chapter 13 (Skin), section 13.4, Topical corticosteroids, Topical corticosteroid preparation potencies

43 B
See BNF, Chapter 3 (Respiratory system), section 3.1.2, Antimuscarinic bronchodilators

44 D
See BNF, Chapter 10 (Musculoskeletal and joint diseases), section 10.1.1, Non-steroidal anti-inflammatory drugs, naproxen

45 E
See BNF, Chapter 10 (Musculoskeletal and joint diseases), section 10.1.4, Gout and cytotoxic-induced hyperuricaemia, Long-term control of gout, Allopurinol

46 C
See BNF, Chapter 2 (Cardiovascular system), section 2.10.2, Fibrinolytic drugs

47 D
See BNF, Chapter 2 (Cardiovascular system), section 2.6.2, Calcium-channel blockers

48 D
See BNF, Chapter 2 (Cardiovascular system), section 2.2.5, Osmotic diuretics

49 E
See BNF, Chapter 13 (Skin), section 13.4, Topical corticosteroids, hydrocortisone, Proprietary hydrocortisone preparations, hydrocortisone

50 E
Infectious diseases which may pose a public health risk must be reported immediately to the appropriate persons. See BNF, Chapter 5 (Infections), Notifiable diseases

51 D
Coronary artery disease is a form of cardiovascular disease.

52 D
See BNF, Chapter 13 (Skin), section 13.10.2, Antifungal preparations, undecenoates

53 C
See BNF, Chapter 4 (Central nervous system), section 4.8.1, Control of the epilepsies, valproic acid

54 E
Fleet Ready-to-use Enema is the only osmotic laxative, the remaining options are all stimulant laxatives. See BNF, Chapter 1 (Gastro-intestinal system), section 1.6.4, Osmotic laxatives, phosphate (rectal)

55 C
See BNF, Chapter 4 (Central nervous system), section 4.3.1, Tricyclic and related antidepressant drugs, Tricyclic antidepressants, amitriptyline hydrochloride

56 B
See BNF, Chapter 5 (Infections), section 5.4.1, Antimalarials, Specific recommendations, North Africa, the Middle East, and Central Asia, Low risk

57 E
Blacklisted preparations are indicated by ~~NHS~~ next to the preparation's name in the BNF or, for an up-to-date list please see latest Drug Tariff. See BNF, Chapter 4 (Central nervous system), section 4.7.1, Non-opioid analgesics and compound analgesic preparations, paracetamol (Acetaminophen)

58 D
See BNF, Emergency treatment of poisoning, Noxious gases

59 C
See BNF, Chapter 14 (Immunological products and vaccines), section 14.4, Vaccines and antisera, Cholera vaccine

MULTIPLE COMPLETION ANSWERS

1 B
See BNF, Chapter 1 (Gastro-intestinal system), section 1.5

2 A
See BNF, Chapter 1 (Gastro-intestinal system), section 1.1.1

3 D
See BNF, Chapter 1 (Gastro-intestinal system), section 1.1.1

4 C
See BNF, Chapter 2 (Cardiovascular system), sections 2.8.1, 2.12 and Chapter 10 (Musculoskeletal and joint diseases), section 10.1.3

5 A
See BNF, Chapter 2 (Cardiovascular system), section 2.10.1

6 D
See BNF, Chapter 2 (Cardiovascular system), section 2.8.1

7 A
See BNF, Chapter 2 (Cardiovascular system), section 2.1.2

8 B
See BNF, Chapter 5 (Infections), section 5.1.12 and Chapter 10 (Musculoskeletal and joint diseases), section 10.1.3

9 A
See BNF, Chapter 3 (Respiratory system), section 3.1

10 D
See BNF, Chapter 4 (Central nervous system), section 4.7.4.1

11 A
See BNF, Chapter 4 (Central nervous system), section 4.8.1

12 B
See BNF, Chapter 4 (Central nervous system), sections 4.3.3 and 4.3.4

13 D
See BNF, Chapter 4 (Central nervous system), section 4.4

14 A
See BNF, Chapter 4 (Central nervous system), section 4.6, Other vestibular disorders

15 A

16 D
See BNF, Appendix 1

17 A
See BNF, Chapter 5 (Infections), section 5.1.7

18 A
See BNF, Chapter 5 (Infections), section 5.1.5

19 A
See BNF, Chapter 5 (Infections), section 5.1.1

20 B

21 C

22 A
See BNF, Chapter 5 (Infections), section 5.3.4

23 D
See BNF, Chapter 6 (Endocrine system), section 6.1.2.1

24 B
See BNF, Chapter 5 (Infections), section 5.3.2

25 A
See BNF, Chapter 6 (Endocrine system), section 6.1.2.3

26 A
See BNF, Chapter 5 (Infections), section 5.2.1 and Chapter 7 (Obstetrics, gynaecology, and urinary-tract disorders), section 7.2.2

27 C
See BNF, Chapter 7 (Obstetrics, gynaecology, and urinary-tract disorders), sections 7.1.1 and 7.1.2

28 C
See BNF, Chapter 7 (Obstetrics, gynaecology, and urinary-tract disorders), section 7.1.3

29 B
See BNF, Chapter 8 (Malignant disease and immunosuppression), section 8.2.4

30 A

31 A
See BNF, Chapter 4 (Central nervous system), section 4.7.3

32 A
See BNF, Chapter 9 (Nutrition and blood), section 9.6.4

33 A
See BNF, Chapter 10 (Musculoskeletal and joint diseases), section 10.1.3

34 A
See BNF, Chapter 11 (Eye), section 11.8.2

35 C
See BNF, Chapter 11 (Eye), section 11.9

36 A
See BNF, Chapter 11 (Eye), sections 11.1 and 11.9

37 A
See BNF, Chapter 11 (Eye), section.11.8.2

38 B
See BNF, Chapter 12 (Ear, nose and oropharynx), section 12.2

39 B
See BNF, Chapter 12 (Ear, nose and oropharynx), section 12.2.2

40 A
See BNF, Chapter 13 (Skin), section 13.5.2

41 D
See BNF, Chapter 13 (Skin), section 13.5.2

42 A
See BNF, Chapter 13 (Skin), section 13.5.2

43 A
See BNF, Chapter 14 (Immunological products and vaccines), section 14.4

44 B
See BNF, Chapter 14 (Immunological products and vaccines), section 14.1

45 B
See BNF, Chapter 14 (Immunological products and vaccines), section 14.1

46 E
See BNF, Chapter 14 (Immunological products and vaccines), section 14.1, Immunisation Schedule

47 A
See BNF, Chapter 15 (Anaesthesia), section 15.1.2

48 A

49 C

50 A
See BNF, Chapter 3 (Respiratory system), section 3.4.3

51 A
See BNF, Chapter 3 (Respiratory system), section 3.4.3

52 A
See BNF, Emergency treatment of poisoning

CLASSIFICATION ANSWERS

1 C
See BNF, Chapter 9 (Nutrition and blood), section 9.2.2

2 D
See BNF, Chapter 10 (Musculoskeletal and joint diseases), section 10.1.3

3 E
See BNF, Chapter 10 (Musculoskeletal and joint diseases), section 10.1.3

4 A
See BNF, Chapter 10 (Musculoskeletal and joint diseases), section 10.1.4

5 A
See BNF, Chapter 10 (Musculoskeletal and joint diseases), section 10.1.4

6 B
See BNF, Chapter 10 (Musculoskeletal and joint diseases), section 10.1.3

7 E
See BNF, Chapter 10 (Musculoskeletal and joint diseases), section 10.1.3

8 D
See BNF, Chapter 10 (Musculoskeletal and joint diseases), section 10.1.3

9 E
See BNF, Chapter 10 (Musculoskeletal and joint diseases), section 10.1.3

10 B
See BNF, Chapter 10 (Musculoskeletal and joint diseases), section 10.1.3

11 E
See BNF, Chapter 5 (Infections), section 5.3.1

12 D
See BNF, Chapter 5 (Infections), section 5.1.1

13 B
See BNF, Chapter 4 (Central nervous system), section 4.9.3

14 B
See BNF, Chapter 4 (Central nervous system), section 4.9.4

15 A
See BNF, Chapter 4 (Central nervous system), section 4.9.1

16 A
See BNF, Chapter 4 (Central nervous system), section 4.9.1

17 C
See BNF, Chapter 4 (Central nervous system), section 4.3.3

18 C
See BNF, Chapter 4 (Central nervous system), section 4.3.3

19 D
See BNF, Chapter 5 (Infections), section 5.1.1

20 C
See BNF, Chapter 4 (Central nervous system), section 4.3.3

21 C
See BNF, Chapter 5 (Infections), section 5.1

22 A
See BNF, Chapter 5 (Infections), section 5.1

23 D
See BNF, Chapter 5 (Infections), section 5.1

24 E
See BNF, Chapter 5 (Infections), section 5.1

25 E
See BNF, Chapter 5 (Infections), section 5.1

26 A
See BNF, Chapter 5 (Infections), section 5.1

27 A
See BNF, Chapter 5 (Infections), section 5.1

28 E
See BNF, Chapter 5 (Infections), section 5.1

29 D
See BNF, Chapter 5 (Infections), section 5.1

30 A
See BNF, Chapter 5 (Infections), section 5.1

31 A
See BNF, Chapter 5 (Infections), section 5.1

32 A
See BNF, Appendix 3

33 E
See BNF, Appendix 3

34 B
See BNF, Appendix 3

35 C
See BNF, Appendix 3

36 D
See BNF, Appendix 3

37 A
See BNF, Appendix 3

38 C
See BNF, Appendix 3

39 B
See BNF, Appendix 3

40 E
See BNF, Appendix 3

41 B
See BNF, Appendix 3

42 B

43 A

44 B

45 B

46 B

47 B

48 C

49 D

50 B

51 E

STATEMENT ANSWERS

1 A
See BNFC, Chapter 5 (Infections), section 5.1.2

2 A
See BNFC, Chapter 5 (Infections), section 5.5.1

3 C
The appropriate dose for a child with a body surface area of 0.5 m^2 or less should be 1.5 mcg/kg three times a week.

4 B
See BNFC, Appendix 2.6

5 B
See BNFC, Chapter 7 (Obstetrics, gynaecology, and urinary-tract disorders), section 7.3

6 C
A dose of 0.01 units/kg/hour is recommended for neonates in intensive care. See BNFC, Chapter 6 (Endocrine system), section 6.1.1

7 B
See BNF, Chapter 5 (Infections), section 5.1.7

8 D
See BNF, Chapter 4 (Central nervous system), section 4.7.4

9 B
See BNF, Chapter 2 (Cardiovascular system), section 2.5.5.1

10 E
Extrapyramidal side-effects reported in neonates when taken in the third trimester See BNF, Chapter 4 (Central nervous system), section 4.2.2

11 E

Roflumilast is licensed as an adjunct to bronchodilators for the maintenance treatment of patients with severe chronic obstructive pulmonary disease associated with chronic bronchitis and a history of exacerbations. See BNF, Chapter 3 (Respiratory system), section 3.3.3

12 B

See BNF, Chapter 10 (Musculoskeletal and joint diseases), section 10.1.1, Non-steroidal anti-inflammatory drugs, Mefenamic acid

13 C

See BNF, Chapter 8 (Malignant disease and immunosuppression), section 8.1.3, Antimetabolites, Pemetrexed

14 C

Application of acaricides following a hot bath is not recommended as it has been shown to increase absorption into the blood and therefore increases risk of adverse systemic effects. See BNF, Chapter 13 (Skin), section 13.10.4, Parasiticidal preparations, Scabies

15 B

Sedating antihistamines have significant antimuscarinic activity and similar adverse effects to antimuscarinic agents. They should therefore be used with caution in patients with prostatic hypertrophy, susceptibility to angle-closure glaucoma, urinary retention and pyloroduodenal obstruction. See BNF, Chapter 3 (Respiratory system), section 3.4.1, Antihistamines

16 B

See BNF, Chapter 2 (Cardiovascular system), section 2.2.1, Thiazides and related diuretics, Indapamide, Modified release

17 B

See BNF, Chapter 9 (Nutrition and blood), section 9.5.5, Selenium

18 B

See BNF, Chapter 2 (Cardiovascular system), section 2.8.1, Parenteral anticoagulants

19 A
See BNF, Chapter 5 (Infections) Notifiable diseases. For further information see Public Health England link available online at: http://www.hpa.org.uk/Topics/InfectiousDiseases/InfectionsAZ/NotificationsOfInfectiousDiseases/ListOfNotifiableDiseases/

20 B
See BNF, Appendix 4 (Intravenous additives), Use of table, Table of drugs given by intravenous infusion, Dopamine hydrochloride

21 A
See BNF, Chapter 4 (Central nervous system), section 4.7.1, Non-opioid analgesics and compound analgesic preparations, Aspirin (Acetylsalicylic Acid), With metoclopramide

22 B
See BNF, Chapter 5 (Infections), section 5.1.13, Urinary-tract infections, nitrofurantoin. See also Appendix 3 (Cautionary and advisory labels for dispensed medicines), Product Label List

23 C
See BNF, Chapter 15 (Anaesthesia), section 15.2, Local anaesthesia, Tetracaine, Tetracaine (Amethocaine). See also Index of manufacturers

24 D
See BNF, Chapter 11 (Eye), section 11.8.1, Tear deficiency, ocular lubricants, and astringents, Sodium Hyaluronate, *Hylo-Care*

25 C
See BNF, Appendix 5 (Wound management products and elasticated garments), section A5.3.4, Other antimicrobials

26 B
See BNF, Chapter 4 (Central nervous system), section 4.7.2, Opioid analgesics, Morphine salts, Oral solutions. See also Appendix 1 (Interactions), List of drug interactions, Analgesics, Opioid Analgesics

27 B
See BNF, Chapter 8 (Malignant disease and immunosuppression), section 8.1.3, Antimetabolites. See also Appendix 1 (Interactions), List of drug interactions, Aminosalicylates

28 A
See BNF, Chapter 8 (Malignant disease and immunosuppression), section 8.1.5, Other antineoplastic drugs, Mitotane. See also Guidance on prescribing, Adverse reactions to drugs

29 B
See BNF, Chapter 4 (Central nervous system), section 4.1.1, Hypnotics

30 B
See BNF, Nurse Prescribers' Formulary, Medicinal preparations

31 D
See BNF, Guidance on prescribing, Emergency supply of medicines, Emergency supply requested by prescriber

32 B
See BNF, Appendix 2 (Borderline substances), section A2.5.1, Special additives for conditions of intolerance

33 D
See BNF, Appendix 4 (Intravenous additives), Use of table, Table of drugs given by intravenous infusion, Tacrolimus

34 C
See BNF, Appendix 2 (Borderline substances), section A2.1.1.1, Enteral feeds: 1 kcal/mL and less than 5 g protein/100 mL, Soya protein formula

35 C
See BNF, Chapter 7 (Obstetrics, gynaecology, and urinary-tract disorders), section 7.3.1, Combined hormonal contraceptives, Combined oral contraceptives, Oral (low and standard strength), Ethinylestradiol with Norethisterone

36 A
See BNF, Appendix 1, Drug interactions

37 B
See BNF, Guidance on prescribing, Prescribing in palliative care, Symptom control

38 C
See BNF, Guidance on prescribing, Prescribing in palliative care, Symptom control

39 D
See BNF, Chapter 11 (Eye), section 11.2, Control of microbial contamination

40 B
See BNF, Guidance on prescribing, Emergency supply of medicines, Emergency supply requested by prescriber

41 B
See BNF, Chapter 13 (Skin), section 13.9, Shampoos and other preparations for scalp and hair conditions, Hirsutism

42 A
See BNF, Dental Practitioners' Formulary, List of dental preparations

43 A
See BNF, Chapter 11 (Eye), section 11.5, Mydriatics and cycloplegics

44 D
See BNF, Chapter 12 (Ear, nose, and oropharynx), section 12.2.2, Topical nasal decongestants

45 B
See MEP, Chapter 3, section 3.3.5, Prescriptions from the EEA or Switzerland, List of EEA countries

46 D
See BNF, Appendix, Dental Practitioners' Formulary, List of Dental Preparations

47 A
See BNF, Chapter 13 (Skin), section 13.2.1.1, Emollient bath and shower preparations

48 D
See BNF, Chapter 11 (Eye), section 11.8.2, Ocular diagnostic and peri-operative preparations and photodynamic treatment, Subfoveal choroidal neovascularisation, ranibizumab and Guidance on prescribing, Adverse reactions to drugs

49 C
Pyridoxine; Vitamin B_6 is used as a prophylactic regimen in patients who are taking isoniazid and are at risk of developing peripheral neuropathy. See BNF, Chapter 5 (Infections), section 5.1.9 Antituberculosis drugs, Isoniazid.

50 C
Alcoholic solutions or suntan lotions must not be used on jellyfish stings as they cause further discharge of the stinging hairs (See BNF, Emergency treatment of poisoning, Other poisons, Marine stings)

51 C
See BNF, Prescribing in palliative care, Pain, Pain management with opioids, Transdermal route

52 C
Heparin and low molecular weight heparins (LMWH) do not cross the placenta. However, they can cause maternal osteoporosis after prolonged use and some multidose vials contain benzyl alcohol which has been associated with fatal toxic syndrome in preterm neonates. See BNF, Chapter 2 (Cardiovascular system), section 2.8.1, Parenteral anticoagulants, Pregnancy. Also, Guidance on prescribing, General guidance, Excipients

53 E
Calcium Resonium is indicated for patients with hyperkalaemia in certain circumstances. Effervescent potassium tablets BPC 1968 do not contain chloride ions and are only used in patients with hyperchloraemia. See BNF, Chapter 9 (Nutrition and blood), section 9.2.1.1, Oral potassium

54 C
See BNF, Chapter 9 (Nutrition and blood), section 9.8.2, Acute porphyrias, Drugs unsafe for use in acute porphyrias, Unsafe Drug Groups

55 B
See BNF, Chapter 13 (Skin), section 13.6.2, Oral preparations for acne, Hormone treatment for acne

56 D
See BNF, Chapter 5 (Infections), section 5.1, Antibacterial drugs, Table 1. Summary of antibacterial therapy, Urinary tract, acute pyelonephritis. See also section 5.1.12, Quinolones, Cautions

57 D
See BNF, Chapter 2 (Cardiovascular system), section 2.2.1, Thiazides and related diuretics

58 B
See BNF, Chapter 5 (Infections), section 5.1.4, Aminoglycosides, gentamicin

59 A
See BNFC, Chapter 2 (Cardiovascular system), section 2.3.2 Drugs for arrhythmias, amiodarone hydrochloride. See also General guidance, excipients

BNF FOR CHILDREN (BNFC) ANSWERS

1 D

2 A
None are licensed for use in children under the age of 1; although they are given at times

3 A

4 A

5 C
See BNFC, Chapter 3 (Respiratory system), section 3.1

6 D
See BNFC, Chapter 8 (Malignant disease and immunosuppression), section 8.1.2

7 A
See BNFC, Chapter 8 (Malignant disease and immunosuppression), section 8.1.1

8 C
See BNFC, Chapter 5 (Infections), section 5.1.9

9 A
See BNFC, Chapter 4 (Central nervous system), section 4.2.1

10 E
See BNFC, Chapter 4 (Central nervous system), section 4.8.1

11 D
Acute pyelonephritis in children over 3 months can be treated with a first-generation cephlasporin or co-amoxiclav for 7–10 days. See BNFC, Chapter 5 (Infections), section 5.1.13

12 E
Vasopressin is not licensed for use in children. See under each drug monograph in BNFC

13 A
See BNFC, Chapter 4, sections 4.9.1, 4.1.1 and BNFC, Chapter 3, Section 3.4.3

14 A
See BNFC, Chapter 8 (Malignant disease and immunosuppression), section 8.2.1

15 A
See BNFC, Chapter 4 (Central nervous system), section 4.7.4.2

16 B
See BNFC, Chapter 9 (Nutrition and blood), section 9.2

17 C
See BNFC, Chapter 2 (Cardiovascular system), section 2.2.2

18 E
See BNFC, Chapter 9 (Nutrition and blood), section 9.1.4

19 E
See BNFC, Chapter 5 (Infections), section 5.1.4 (2.5 mg/kg = 2.5 mg × 2 kg = 5 mg)

20 D
0.46

21 A
See BNFC, Chapter 2 (Cardiovascular system), section 2.14

22 D
See BNFC, Chapter 3 (Respiratory system), section 3.1

23 C
See BNFC, Chapter 5 (Infections), section 5.4.1

24 B
See BNFC, Chapter 1 (Gastro-intestinal system), section 1.3

25 D
See BNFC, Chapter 2 (Cardiovascular system), section 2.5

26 B
See BNFC, Chapter 13 (Skin), section 13.10.3

27 A
See BNFC, Chapter 5 (Infections), section 5.1.1.1

28 A
See BNFC, Chapter 5 (Infections), section 5.1.1.1

29 C
See BNFC, Chapter 5 (Infections), section 5.1.8

30 C
See BNFC, Chapter 5 (Infections), section 5.1.8

Closed book answers

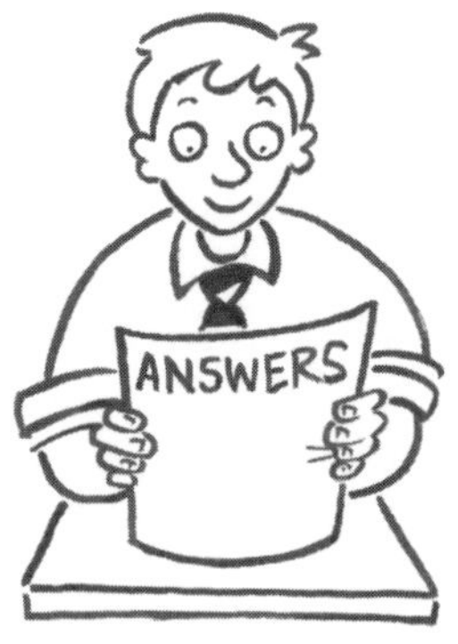

SIMPLE COMPLETION ANSWERS

1 D

2 B
'Missed pill' is one that is 24 hours late

3 C
OTC treatments for cystitis containing sodium citrate should not be sold for patients with hypertension; to men under any circumstances; to patients taking lithium because sodium is preferentially absorbed by the kidney, increasing the excretion of lithium and resulting in reduced plasma lithium concentrations; to pregnant women. There is no contraindication or interaction with levodopa

4 B
Hydrocortisone cream is licensed for use in children of 10 years and over; chloramphenicol eye ointment is licensed only for the treatment of acute bacterial conjunctivitis; diclofenac is licensed for other types of pain as well as muscular and rheumatic, as well as for colds, influenza and fever; amoxicillin is not licensed for non-prescription sale

5 E
Potentially hazardous pharmacodynamic interactions have been identified between triptans and St John's wort, leading to an increased risk of adverse effects

6 B
See BNF, Appendix 3

7 C
Prochlorperazine is licensed for non-prescription sale only for the treatment of nausea and vomiting associated with migraine

8 B
Feeling *cold* is a symptom of hypoglycaemia

9 C
Measles shares some of the symptoms described with some of the other conditions listed, but the lesions in the mouth (Koplik's spots) are characteristic.

10 E
Penciclovir cream should be applied every two hours during waking hours, i.e. approximately eight times per day

11 C
GTN tablets should be taken sitting down

12 D
Corticosteroids are used to treat Addison's disease

13 B
This question refers to OTC supply, not prescription (see BNF, section 13.4). It can be sold to treat allergic contact dermatitis, irritant dermatitis, and insect bite reactions and mild to moderate eczema. However it may not be sold to children under 12 or in pregnancy except under medical advice. Contraindications include use on eye or face, anogenital region, broken or infected skin, acne or athletes' foot. Use is restricted to a max. of 1 week.

14 A
See BNF, Chapter 3 (Respiratory system), section 3.1.3

15 B
Oral contraceptive commonly causes migraine

16 C

17 D

18 A

19 D
Loop diuretics cause hypomagnesaemia

20 B

21 D
See BNF, Appendix 3 (Cautionary label 7)

22 E

23 E

24 D

25 A

26 B

27 D

28 D

29 E

30 B

31 C
See Practice Guidance document, Substance of misuse

32 C
See MEP, section 1.2.3, Prescription-only medicines (POM), Emergency supplies of prescription-only medicines

33 D
Methadone is a schedule 2 Controlled Drug which is used to treat opioid misusers and can only be legally prescribed and dispensed against a valid instalment prescription. Pharmacists must be aware of the abuse potential of any Controlled Drug. See MEP, section 1.2.14, Controlled Drugs, National Health prescriptions for the treatment of misusers

34 A
Digoxin is a cardiac glycoside and is a positive ionotrope. It increases the force of contraction of the heart and reduces conductivity in the AV node

35 E
Furosemide is a loop diuretic. One of the side-effects that may occur with furosemide therapy is hypokalaemia. Hypokalaemia predisposes to digoxin toxicity. Therefore, the patient should be monitored for signs of toxicity, such as nausea and bradycardia.

36 D

37 E

38 C
Lithium therapy may cause hyperthyroidism and hyperparathyroidism. For this reason, thyroid function is monitored every 6 months while on lithium therapy. If there is evidence of deterioration of thyroid function, then monitoring may be more frequent than 6 months.

39 A
Naproxen is an NSAID. NSAIDs reduce the excretion of lithium, thereby causing accumulation of the drug leading to an increased risk of lithium toxicity.

40 C
Neuropathic pain occurs as a result of damage to neural tissue. The pain is generally managed with tricyclic antidepressants or antiepileptic drugs. Phenytoin is unlicensed, but is very effective for neuropathic pain.

41 B

42 B
Phenytoin requires therapeutic drug monitoring, as it has a narrow therapeutic index. The desired serum concentration for phenytoin is 10–20 mg/L

43 D
Digoxin is indicated for atrial fibrillation, heart failure and tachycardias

44 C
Professional standards and guidance for the sale and supply of medicines

45 C
ACE I should be initiated under specialist supervision

46 A
GI side-effects are common with metformin and may persist in some patients, therefore the dose is slowly titrated up. See BNF, Chapter 6 (Endocrine system), section 6.1.2

47 B

48 A
Rare reports of liver dysfunction, seek immediate medical attention if signs of liver impairment occur. See BNF, Chapter 6 (Endocrine system), section 6.1.2

49 D

50 E
See BNF, Chapter 7 (Obstetrics, gynaecology, and urinary-tract disorders), section 7.3.1

MULTIPLE COMPLETION ANSWERS

1 B

Enzyme inducers and inhibitors are responsible for important pharmacokinetic interactions which lead to altered drug levels and clinical effect. However, the time it takes for the enzyme inducers and inhibitors to exert their full effects and wear off differs: enzyme inducers (2–3 weeks) and enzyme inhibitors (a few days). This is not always the case, as some enzyme inducers/inhibitors may act faster or slower than others.
Ref: Wiffen, P., Mitchell, M., Snelling, M. and Stoner, N. (2012). *Oxford Handbook of Clinical Pharmacy*, 2nd edition. Oxford: Oxford University Press, Chapter 2, pp. 20, 23

2 A

http://www.nhs.uk/Livewell/alcohol/Pages/alcohol-units.aspx

3 A

See BNF, Guidance on prescribing, Prescribing in renal impairment

4 D

See BNF, Chapter 5 (Infections), section 5.1.12, Quinolones, Cautions. Quinolones have been shown to cause arthropathy in weight-bearing joints of young animals and are therefore cautioned in young children and growing adolescents

5 E

See BNF, Chapter 6 (Endocrine system), section 6.4.1.1, Oestrogens and HRT, Hormone replacement therapy and Contraception. Also Chapter 7 (Obstetrics, gynaecology, and urinary-tract disorders), section 7.3.1, Combined hormonal contraceptives, Reasons to stop immediately

6 A

See MEP, section 2.4, Taking medication histories, Sources of information

7 C

See BNF, Chapter 1 (Gastro-intestinal system), section 1.5, Chronic bowel disorders, *Clostridium difficile* infection

8 A
The strength of hypromellose must be checked with the prescriber before dispensing the product. It is essential that some preparations are specified by brand. This is mainly due to pharmacokinetic or other variations. For example, different theophylline m/r preparations have different absorption rates. Different preparations of nifedipine m/r tablets may not have the same clinical effect. Other formulations which need to be specified by brand name include: beclometasone CFC-free inhalers and lithium, phenytoin and mesalazine preparations. See BNF under 'preparations' for the corresponding medications for further details

9 E
All registered pharmacists are required to complete a minimum of nine entries per year. At least three of these must start with the reflection phase of the CPD cycle. See MEP, section 2.8.1, Continuing professional development, opportunities for CPD

10 A
See BNF, Chapter 10 (Musculoskeletal and joint diseases), section 10.1.1, Non-steroidal anti-inflammatory drugs, Ibuprofen

11 A
See MEP, section 3.2.5, Cough and cold medicines for children

12 B
'Use by' or 'Use before' means that the product in question, may only be used up to the end of the previous month. Expiry date means that the product in question should not be used after the last day of the month stated, unless a specific date is mentioned, See MEP, section 3.5.1, Expiry dates, and section 3.5.2, Waste medicines

13 A
Anxiogenic agents are those which cause anxiety. See, Charney, D.S., Heninger, G.R. and Jatlow, P.I. (1985) 'Increased anxiogenic effects of caffeine in panic disorders.' *Arch. Gen. Psychiatry* 42(3): 233–43. See also, Rogers, P.J., Hohoff, C., Heatherley, S.V., Mullings, E.L., Maxfield, P.J., Evershed, R.P. *et al.* (2010) 'Association of the anxiogenic and alerting effects of caffeine with ADORA2A and ADORA1 polymorphisms and habitual level of caffeine consumption.' *Neuropsychopharmacology* 35(9): 1973–83

14 A
See relevant Responding to Symptoms textbook

15 A
Drugs with a narrow window between therapeutic and toxic dosage ranges include: theophylline, carbamazepine, digoxin, warfarin, lithium, clonidine, phenytoin, prazosin and minoxidil. See Lodola, A. and Stadler, J. (2011) 'Commonly used risk management strategies', in *Pharmaceutical Toxicology in Practice: A Guide to Non-Clinical Development* Wiley-Blackwell, p. 239, table 11.2

16 A
See BNF, Chapter 13 (Skin), section 13.10.4, Parasiticidal preparations, Scabies

17 A
See relevant Responding to Symptoms textbook

18 A
See BNF Guidance on Prescribing, Prescription writing

19 C
See BNF, Chapter 12 (Ear, nose, and oropharynx), section 12.3.1, Drugs for oral ulceration and inflammation, doxycycline, and section 12.3.4, Mouthwashes, gargles, and dentifrices, chlorhexidine gluconate

20 A
See relevant Responding to Symptoms textbook

21 D
A granuloma is a small area of inflammation which results from tissue injury. Cerebral astrocytoma is cancer of the brain and Ewing's sarcoma is cancer of the bone or soft tissue. See relevant Responding to Symptoms textbook

22 B
See MHRA, 'List of substances – List C' available online at: http://www.mhra.gov.uk/Howweregulate/Medicines/Licensingofmedicines/Legalstatusandreclassification/Listsofsubstances/index.htm

23 B
See relevant Responding to Symptoms textbook

24 A
See BNF, Appendix 3 Cautionary and advisory labels for dispensed medicines, labels 5 and 6

25 D
A cryptogenic disease is one in which the cause is unknown. See relevant Responding to Symptoms textbook

26 A
Non-communicable diseases are those which cannot spread between people

27 A
See BNF, Chapter 4 (Central nervous system), section 4.10.3, Opioid dependence, Adjunctive therapy and symptomatic treatment

28 C
See MHRA 'List of substances – List C' available online at: http://www.mhra.gov.uk/Howweregulate/Medicines/Licensingofmedicines/Legalstatusandreclassification/Listsofsubstances/index.htm

29 B
See relevant Responding to Symptoms textbook

30 A
Anorexia nervosa, bulimia nervosa and pica are classified as mental disorders in standard medical manuals such as ICD-10 (available online at: http://priory.com/psych/ICD.htm)

31 B
See BNF, Chapter 7 (Obstetrics, gynaecology, and urinary-tract disorders), section 7.3.5, Emergency contraception, Hormonal methods, Levonorgestrel

32 E
Mesothelioma is a cancer which develops from cells of the mesothelium which commonly affect the pleural lining of the lungs. It is associated with asbestos exposure. See relevant Responding to Symptoms textbook

33 C
Nicotinell lozenges are for those above the age of 18 years. See BNF, Chapter 4 (Central nervous system), section 4.10.2, Nicotine dependence, Nicotine replacement therapy

34 A
See Drug misuse and dependence, UK guidelines on clinical management, available online at: http://www.nta.nhs.uk/uploads/clinical_guidelines_2007.pdf

35 A
See BNF, Chapter 4 (Central nervous system), section 4.10.1, Alcohol dependence

36 D
See BNFC, Chapter 3 (Respiratory system), section 3.4.1, Antihistamines, Non-sedating antihistamines, fexofenadine

37 A
See BNF. Also Appendix 3, Cautionary and advisory labels for dispensed medicines, label 11

38 B
See BNF, Chapter 3 (Respiratory system), section 3.4.3, Allergic emergencies, Anaphylaxis, Adrenaline/epinephrine, Intramuscular injection for self-administration

39 A
See relevant Responding to Symptoms textbook

40 A
See relevant Responding to Symptoms textbook

41 B
Lichen simplex and psoriasis are conditions of the skin which are associated with localised demarcated plaques. *Listeria monocytogenes* is a bacterium which causes listeriosis. See relevant Responding to Symptoms textbook

42 D
See BNF, Chapter 5 (Infections), section 5.1.12, Quinolones

43 B
See BNF individual monographs

44 A
See BNF individual monographs

45 A
See BNF, Chapter 4 (Central nervous system), section 4.7.4.1, Treatment of acute migraine, 5HT1-receptor agonists

46 B
See relevant Responding to Symptoms textbook

47 A
Salicylate-, pseudoephedrine- and codeine-containing products are not suitable for use in pregnant women

48 A
See MHRA, 'Public health risk with herbal medicines: An overview', available online at: http://www.mhra.gov.uk/home/groups/es-herbal/documents/websiteresources/con023163.pdf

49 A
See MHRA, 'List of substances – List C', available online at: http://www.mhra.gov.uk/Howweregulate/Medicines/Licensingofmedicines/Legalstatusandreclassification/Listsofsubstances/index.htm

50 C
See relevant Responding to Symptoms textbook

51 B
See BNF, Chapter 8 (Malignant disease and immunosuppression), section 8.1, Cytotoxic drugs, side-effects of cytotoxic drugs; and section 8.1.1, Alkylating drugs

52 A
See MEP, Appendix 10, GPhC guidance for responsible pharmacists, Displaying the notice; and Appendix B, The notice

53 A
See WHO report, 'Use of Glycated Haemoglobin (HbA1c) in the Diagnosis of Diabetes Mellitus'. Available online at: http://www.who.int/diabetes/publications/report-hba1c_2011.pdf

54 B
See http://www.nhsinform.co.uk/health-library/articles/d/drug-misuse/facts

55 B
People who present with 'alarm features' including bleeding, dysphagia, recurrent vomiting or weight loss must be referred immediately for urgent endoscopic investigation. See BNF, Chapter 1 (Gastro-intestinal system), section 1.1, Dyspepsia and gastro-oesophageal reflux disease, Dyspepsia

56 C
Phenobarbital and midazolam (as well as temazepam and buprenorphine) are CD 3 ('CD No Reg') drugs and are not required to be recorded in the CD register. See MEP, Chapter 3 (Controlled drugs), section 3.7.2, Classification

57 C
See BNF, individual drug monographs

58 B
See advice from Public Health England (formally Health Protection Agency), available online at: http://www.hpa.org.uk/Topics/InfectiousDiseases/InfectionsAZ/Malaria/GeneralInformation/mala10Background/. Or see recommended Responding to Symptoms textbook

59 C
See BNF, General guidance, Extemporaneous preparation

60 E
See MEP, Appendix 10, GPhC guidance for responsible pharmacists, Absence

61 B
See BNF, General Guidance, Safety in the home

62 A
See BNF, How the BNF is constructed, Sources of BNF information

CLASSIFICATION ANSWERS

1 C
See BNF, Chapter5 (Infections), section 5.1.11, metronidazole and tinidazole, metronidazole

2 C
See BNF, Chapter5 (Infections), section 5.1.11, metronidazole and tinidazole, metronidazole

3 E
See BNF, Chapter 4 (Central nervous system), section 4.3.2, monoamine-oxidase inhibitors, moclobemide

4 A
See BNF, Chapter 4 (Central nervous system), section 4.2.3, Antimanic drugs, lithium

5 D
See material safety data sheet 'MSDS', Phenol Liquid

6 E
See BNF, Chapter 13 (Skin), section 13.2.2, Barrier preparations, Proprietary barrier preparations

7 C
See BNF, Chapter 11 (Eye), section 11.8.1, Tear deficiency, ocular lubricants, and astringents, liquid paraffin

8 A
NHS, available online at: http://www.nhs.uk/Conditions/Dehydration/Pages/Symptoms.aspx

9 B
See BNF, Chapter 14 (Immunological products and vaccines), section 14.1, Active immunity, side-effects

10 B
Myocardial infarction is a terminology used for heart attacks

11 A
Shortness of breath (SOB) is a clinical sign also known as dyspnoea

12 D
A cerebrovascular accident (CVA) is a stroke

13 E
Last menstrual period (LMP)
See relevant medical terminology books such as: *Medical Terminology for Health Professions* by Carol L. Schroeder and Ann Ehrlich, and *Medical Terminology Made Incredibly Easy!*, by Springhouse

14 B

15 A

16 C
BNF, Chapter 11 (Eye), section 11.6, Treatment of glaucoma, beta-blockers.

17 E
Hypermetropia is the inability to focus on near objects whereas, myopia is where distant objects appear blurred.
See relevant medical terminology books such as *Medical Terminology for Health Professions*, by Carol L. Schroeder and Ann Ehrlich and *Medical Terminology Made Incredibly Easy!*, by Springhouse.

18 B
A patient who is taking insulin and experiencing hypoglycaemic symptoms requires dose adjustment or change of medication

19 C
Patients (or their carers) who are taking phenytoin must be advised to seek immediate medical attention if symptoms such as fever, rash, mouth ulcers, bruising or bleeding develop. See BNF, Chapter 4 (Central nervous system), section 4.8.1, Control of the epilepsies, Phenytoin 3.

20 B
The patient may require dose adjustment as chronic constipation is a symptom of hypothyroidism

21 E
Warfarin is not commonly associated with constipation.

22 D

23 A

24 B

25 C
Refer to relevant Responding to Symptoms textbook

26 B
See BNF, Chapter 2 (Cardiovascular system), section 2.2.1, Thiazides and related diuretics

27 C
See BNF, Chapter 4 (Central nervous system), section 4.3.3, Selective serotonin re-uptake inhibitors

28 E
See BNF, Chapter 9 (Nutrition and blood), section 9.5.2.2, Phosphate-binding agents

29 A
See BNF, Chapter 10 (Musculoskeletal and joint diseases), section 10.1.3, Drugs that suppress the rheumatic disease process, Cytokine modulators

30 C
See BNF, Chapter 2 (Cardiovascular system), section 2.3.2, Drugs for arrhythmias, supraventricular arrhythmias

31 B
See BNF, Chapter 2 (Cardiovascular system), section 2.11, Antifibrinolytic drugs and haemostatics

32 E
See BNF, Chapter 1 (Gastro-intestinal system), section 1.2, Antispasmodics and other drugs altering gut motility, Other antispasmodics

33 B
See BNF, Emergency treatment of poisoning, Specific drugs

34 D
See BNF, Emergency treatment of poisoning, Specific drugs

35 C
See BNF, Emergency treatment of poisoning, Specific drugs

36 B
See relevant Responding to Symptoms textbook

37 C
See relevant Responding to Symptoms textbook

38 E
See relevant Responding to Symptoms textbook

39 D
See relevant Responding to Symptoms textbook

40 B

41 C

42 A

43 E
See relevant Responding to Symptoms textbook

44 E
See BNF, Chapter 9 (Nutrition and blood), section 9.6.2, Vitamin B group

45 A
See BNF, Chapter 9 (Nutrition and blood), section 9.1.2, Drugs used in megaloblastic anaemias

46 B
See BNF, Chapter 9 (Nutrition and blood), section 9.6.1, Vitamin A; and see BNFC

47 D
See BNF, Chapter 9 (Nutrition and blood), section 9.6.6, Vitamin K

48 B
See BNF, Chapter 9 (Nutrition and blood), section 9.6.2, Vitamin B group

49 D
See BNF, Chapter 9 (Nutrition and blood), section 9.1.2, Drugs used in megaloblastic anaemias

50 C
See BNF, Chapter 9 (Nutrition and blood), section 9.6.2, Vitamin B group, Pyridoxine hydrochloride

51 E
See BNF, Chapter 9 (Nutrition and blood), section 9.6.2, Vitamin B group

52 B

53 A

54 C

55 E
See relevant medical terminology books such as *Medical Terminology for Health Professions*, by Carol L. Schroeder and Ann Ehrlich and *Medical Terminology Made Incredibly Easy!*, by Springhouse

56 C
A haemangioma is a collection of abnormal blood vessels which form a lump in or under the skin.

57 B
Blood following a cough must be referred as a matter of urgency

58 D
Hemiballismus is a rare condition which presents as a violent form of dyskinesia

59 A
Hematochezia is the passage of bright red bloody stools. See NHS choices, available online at: http://www.nhs.uk/Pages/HomePage.aspx; and *Medical Terminology Guide* by Joseph Jakubal

60 A

61 C

62 B

63 E
See inside back cover of BNF, or Latin abbreviations textbook (e.g. *Terminology for Allied Health Professionals*, by C. Sormunen and R.F. Jones

64 B

65 D

66 A

67 E
See relevant medical terminology books such as *Medical Terminology for Health Professions*, by Carol L. Schroeder and Ann Ehrlich, and *Medical Terminology Made Incredibly Easy!*, by Springhouse

68 B
See BNF, Chapter 2 (Cardiovascular system), section 2.9, Antiplatelet drugs, Dipyridamole, With aspirin

69 C
See BNF, Chapter 2 (Cardiovascular system), section 2.12, Lipid-regulating drugs, Statins, simvastatin

70 A
See BNF, Chapter 2 (Cardiovascular system), section 2.6.1, Nitrates

71 D
See BNF, Chapter 6 (Endocrine system), section 6.6.2, Bisphosphonates and other drugs affecting bone metabolism, Bisphosphonates, alendronic acid

72 A

73 D

74 B

75 C
See relevant medical terminology books such as *Medical Terminology for Health Professions*, by Carol L. Schroeder and Ann Ehrlich, and *Medical Terminology Made Incredibly Easy!*, by Springhouse

76 C
See BNF, Chapter 3 (Respiratory system), section 3.1.2, Antimuscarinic bronchodilators, Ipratropium bromide

77 A
See BNF, Chapter 2 (Cardiovascular system), section 2.5.5.1, Angiotensin-converting enzyme inhibitors, ramipril

78 D
See BNF, Chapter 4 (Central nervous system), section 4.2.1, Antipsychotic drugs, Second-generation antipsychotic drugs, olanzapine

79 E
See BNF, Chapter 4 (Central nervous system), section 4.8.1, Control of the epilepsies, Carbamazepine and related antiepileptics, carbamazepine

STATEMENT QUESTIONS

1 B
See MEP, section 2.8

2 E
The age of the patient if under 12 years old is a legal requirement, see MEP, section 3.3

3 E
Repeatable prescriptions can only be dispensed against a private prescription. If the quantity of repeat is not stated, then it can only be repeated once, see MEP, section 3.3.1

4 B
See MEP, section 3.3.3

5 C
See MEP, section 3.3.5, Turkey is not in the EEA

6 C
See MEP, section 3.3.10.2

7 C
See MEP, section 3.5.10

8 D
See MEP, section 3.6

9 E
See MEP, section 3.7.2

10 B
See MEP, section 3.7.6

11 C
Hypokalaemia predisposes the patient to digoxin toxicity. Digoxin does not cause hypokalaemia as a side-effect

12 B
Both are side-effects of the drug but have no relation to each other

13 B
See BNF, Chapter 2 (Cardiovascular system)

14 A
See BNF, Appendix 1

15 C
See BNF, Chapter 1 (Gastro-intestinal system), section 1.3

16 A
See BNF, Chapter 2 (Cardiovascular system), section 2.6.3

17 C
See BNF, Chapter 2 (Cardiovascular system), section 2.5.5

18 A
See BNF, Chapter 5 (Infections), section 5.1.12

19 A
Hyponatraemia has been associated with antidepressant therapy. If patients develop drowsiness, convulsions or confusion, hyponatraemia should be considered as convulsions are a symptom of hyponatraemia
See BNF, Chapter 4 (Central nervous system), sections 4.3 and 4.3.3

20 C
See BNF, Chapter 3 (Respiratory system), section 3.1.1.1

21 D
See BNF, Chapter 4 (Central nervous system), section 4.2.1

22 A
See BNF, Chapter 4 (Central nervous system), section 4.3.2

23 A
See BNF, Chapter 5 (Infections), section 5.1.1.2

24 B
See BNF, Chapter 5 (Infections), section 5.1.6 and section 5.1, Table 1

25 D
See BNF, Chapter 6 (Endocrine system), section 6.1.2.2

26 B
See BNF, Chapter 6 (Endocrine system), section 6.3.2

27 B
See BNF, Chapter 6 (Endocrine system), section 6.4.2

28 A
See BNF, Chapter 9 (Nutrition and blood), section 4.9.2

29 C
See BNF, Chapter 4 (Central nervous system), section 4.2.3. Hyponatraemia predisposes to lithium toxicity so patients should maintain adequate salt intake

30 A
See BNF, Chapter 6 (Endocrine system), section 6.1.2.2

31 A
See BNF, Chapter 6 (Endocrine system), section 6.6.2

32 D
See BNF, Chapter 4 (Central nervous system), section 4.7.2. Diamorphine is a schedule 2 controlled drug.

33 C
See BNF, Appendix 1. Antihypertensives and sympathomimetics can cause severe hypertension when given together

34 D
See BNF, Chapter 13 (Skin), section 13.4

35 B
See BNF, Chapter 2 (Cardiovascular system), section 2.8.2

36 A
See BNF, Appendix 1

37 B
See BNF, Chapter 2 (Cardiovascular system), section 2.2.2

38 B
See BNF, Chapter 3 (Respiratory system), section 3.4.1

39 D
See BNF, Chapter 4 (Central nervous system), section 4.1.2

40 B
See BNF, Chapter 4 (Central nervous system), section 4.6

Index